About Dr. Slack

Robert Slack spent his boyhood in Helena, Montana. At age fourteen, his family moved to Hawaii where his father, Howard Slack, became Hawaii's first federal veterinarian at the time of statehood in 1959. After graduating from Kailua High School on Oahu, Bob attended Washington State University graduating with honors from the College of Veterinary Medicine in 1971. Pursuing his passion for adventure, he moved to Australia to begin his veterinary career, first in Sydney, and later in Perth. After several years abroad, Bob returned to the U.S. to join a small animal practice in Spokane, Washington. Mid career he returned to college to pursue his interest in human behavioral science, and earned a degree in counseling.

The blending of these two careers, both full time in veterinary medicine and part time in counseling, has given Bob a rich and unique perspective in writing this book on the miracle of the human-animal bond.

Tails

Curious Stories Of The Human-Animal Bond

...

Robert Slack, DVM

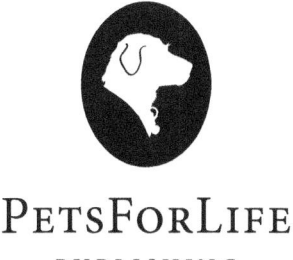

PetsForLife
PUBLISHING

P.O. Box 497
Colbert, WA 99005-0497
www.petsforlife.com

FIRST EDITION | PETSFORLIFE PUBLISHING | JUNE 2017

ISBN: 978-0-578-19305-2
Copyright © 2017 by Robert Slack, DVM

All rights reserved. No part of this publication may be reproduced, distributed, or transmitted in any form or by any means, including photocopying, recording, or other electronic or mechanical methods, without the prior written permission of the publisher, except in the case of brief quotations embodied in critical reviews and certain other noncommercial uses permitted by copyright law.
For permission requests, write to the publisher, at the address below.

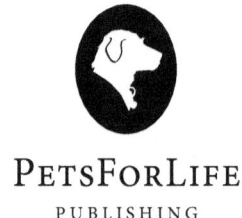

PETSFORLIFE
PUBLISHING

P.O. Box 497
COLBERT, WA 99005-0497
info@petsforlife.com

Ordering Information: www.petsforlife.com.
Quantity Sales–Special discounts are available on quantity purchases by corporations, associations, schools, and others.
For details, contact the publisher at the address above.

Printed in South Korea

Memorium

In memory of J. Howard Slack D.V.M.
a devoted father, dedicated veterinarian, and community servant.

Foreword

Gratitude, resonance and admiration are the key words that come to mind when I try to characterize my journey with Dr. Bob Slack as we followed the path toward the full realization of his book, Tails.

In a world filled with seemingly endless distractions and demands on our time, those of us with pets, especially dogs and cats, know the joy of coming home to wildly wagging tails and the loving greetings they so unfailingly give us each time we enter the house. These moments embody the enduring and universal messages found in this book: pets are our friends, our playmates, our confidants and our teachers. They help us diminish the sense of pressure or strain that our life responsibilities and personal technology devices often place on us. So for us pet lovers, rather than get excessively involved in "Tweets" and "likes", we have chosen instead the paws and licks of our pets as a means of relaxing and feeling the benefits of "the bond" that Dr. Slack so movingly describes throughout this book.

My relationship with Dr. Bob has spanned 18 years. He cared for my Westies (Bizzy and Pookee) from their very first puppy checkups, until the twilight years of their lives. They actually liked going to the vet's office…no matter what miscellaneous parts might have been missing when they returned home. Early on, his advanced surgical abilities were called upon with each dog. First, money hungry dog, Bizzy, had eaten two quarters which had ultimately fused together and became lodged in his upper intestines. Dr. Bob had to surgically remove them. Then, shortly after, came the big jolt…he found and removed a cancerous tumor from Pookee's lower intestines.

Here is where the key word of "gratitude" kicks in. I am and will forever be grateful for Dr. Slack's exceptional diagnostic and surgical skills. During a post-op visit he had arranged for us at Washington State University's Veterinarian Oncology department, Pookee had a full day of thorough follow-up tests so we could determine appropriate further treatments to ensure, as best we could, that his cancer was eradicated. Imagine my relief and elation when the doctors thought the best course was to skip radiation and chemotherapy entirely, and just keep a close eye on things going forward. Why? They determined Dr. Slack's early detection and surgical intervention had prevented an otherwise malignant cancer from spreading. Their tests revealed no evidence of cancer remaining in the surgical margins and Pookee was allowed to live out his life to a full Westie age, all cancer free.

It was sometime a few years later, during a routine office visit with both of the Westies, that Dr. Bob casually mentioned he was considering writing a book on his lifetime of observing the nature and mystery of the deep and wonderful "bond" that we as humans share with our pets, despite the vast differential in our respective life spans. I was intrigued immediately. Within my thoughts, I could feel a strong resonance (another key word) had occurred for me upon hearing his premise and the associated ideas and experiences supporting it.

The timing was also fortuitous, as I had just recently retired as a global marketing director for one of the industry groups at an international management consulting corporation. One aspect *of my career, for the past 17 years, had centered on communications, publishing articles & brochures and structuring thematic story lines for large executive conferences. Consequently, I still carried the ingrained habit of always being on the lookout for knowledgeable, interesting people with unique perspectives and fresh, insightful messages to invite as speakers or as collaborators at conferences or writing articles. Though I am retired now and no longer produce events, I know a good story when I hear it.* Tails *is a good story!*

So, resonance – Bob's story ideas were extraordinarily powerful to me and his style of telling them was filled with humor, while being mindful of both pet and human fragilities. They were based in the science and medical training he rigorously followed in keeping our pets healthy, as well as deep compassion for the human condition. Bob's concern for the people-side of the equation was amplified by his background in counseling. Mid-career he took leave of his veterinary practice to pursue credentials in counseling and then worked with individuals struggling with drug addiction before returning full time to his veterinary profession. The synergy of these two career paths becomes evident as he writes of a man in the early stages of recovery whose bond with his pet gave him the strength to risk re-entering the human world – yet another gift of the human-animal bond.

During his early writing process, we would periodically meet for lunch to discuss various ideas about the potential value of writing such a book, who might like to read it and options for how it could be structured. Occasionally, he would send me an example chapter or two to test a concept. Unfailingly, upon reading them, I would be mesmerized and moved by the power of the situations he had experienced and the amusing writing style he used to describe his observations.

At that point I had only seen five or six standalone, random chapters. But later, when I read his fully fleshed-out manuscript for the first time, I was utterly astonished by both its intense emotional impact and its positive affirmation of humanity. Seeing the book as a whole left me speechless. It was a love story…love shared between a pet and their human, as well as with a caring, skilled vet to support and extend this love affair. Clearly, this was a book that I believed needed to be written and would be greatly appreciated by the multiple audiences of pet lovers, veterinary students, mental health counselors, people seeking spiritual insights on lifecycle matters and good old-fashioned book aficionados looking for a well written, humorous read.

Dr. Bob's own personal career journey, which is another fascinating aspect of Tails, *is laid open and made visible as a tale of its own. His powerful vignettes tell of life through the lens of a veterinarian – the person to whom we entrust the wellbeing of our beloved pets. It is this perspective that makes* Tails *so captivating, because his stories allow us to enter into a world that is dominated by pets and the people who love them…and who sooner or later, grieve for them.*

He tells in rich, vivid detail about some of his most touching, demanding or hilarious office experiences and elegantly transforms them into compelling and engaging stories – each one reflecting his ability to seamlessly conjoin medical sciences with his deep empathy for people and their love of animal companions. Every story is made easily accessible to us non-veterinarians through his perceptive telling of the profound life moments we experience with our pets – often times laugh-out-loud funny, sometimes emotionally poignant, but always entertaining with a sly linguistic wit. His stories make detectable the subtle irony that some of the most human of spiritual lessons can emerge from our involvement with four-legged, animal friends.

Tails is a powerful and affecting read. If you love dogs or cats, I doubt you will be able to put it down once you start reading it, because the overall reading experience is so exhilarating and uplifting. Each of the times I have read and re-read the book, my response was the same. I was spellbound! Each time I was pulled into his world so completely that I read it straight through in one sitting. Each time I felt deeply enriched from the book's messages and became increasingly aware of an expansion of my spirit. I appreciated in new and more complete ways all of the dogs I have had during my lifetime and how special they were in creating a sense of wellbeing and joy. I hold great admiration (final key word) of Dr. Slack's talent for weaving a broad range of topics into cohesive stories spanning the lifecycle of our pets…and of us humans; all of which is told in a manner that reads like a page-turner novel.

I predict you too will be hooked on this book from the first to the last page. You will smile often, maybe even laugh out loud, perhaps find tears welling up in your eyes at times, and above all, feel a joyful, enriched awareness of the precious gift we have in our relationship with pets as seen through the eyes of the author. Tails is a serious book written in a light-hearted yet enlightening style. It makes you think. It makes you feel. It makes you grateful and consciously appreciative of the existence of pets in our lives.

I feel blessed to have been a small part of the journey with this amazing gentleman – a journey from a casual remark to a finished book.

February 2017

JIM SAYLES
Spokane, Washington

Acknowledgements

I am forever indebted to my professors for their resolute efforts to instill in me the knowledge and skills necessary to be worthy of the title: veterinarian. And to respect the Hippocratic Oath: "Do no Harm".

To all those people, both clients and friends, who shared stories of the many ways pets enriched their lives. It gave me a wonderful portal to witness the human-animal bond – and to my own pets for their companionship from boyhood to old age.

My heartfelt appreciation to my wife, Lois, for her patience, encouraging words, and helpful suggestions in bringing this book to fruition and to my children who insisted we never be without a pet to protect them from things that go bump in the night.

A special thanks to Patrick Cotter for his perceptive edits and for teaching me the invaluable lesson of knowing what to leave out. To Terry Mitchell for her insistence that the written language be treated respectfully and to Janice Strong for her courage to venture into Tails to administer editing resuscitation.

Dr. Linda Lee Wood, a respected colleague and friend, has given me helpful insight coming from her many years as a successful small animal clinician – she is no stranger to the human-animal bond.

My thanks to Dr. Paul Quinnett, an accomplished writer and sportsman, for reading my manuscript and giving me helpful suggestions. And to Sharon Wegscheider-Cruse, author and storyteller, thank you for your encouraging words. You gave me direction when I needed it most.

To Deanna Camp for her expertise and dedication in taking on the task of graphic design, illustration, copywriting, and managing the complicated process of moving a manuscript draft to a finished book – along with her daughter Ruby, who gave it a once-over for grammar.

I would be sorely remiss to not include Jim Sayles. He trusted me with the health of his pets and gave unselfishly of his time, advice and encouragement in taking the next step in publishing my work. He penned the Forward to Tails.

The names of my clients and their pets have been changed for the writing of this book in order to protect their identities.

Contents

Prologue	xix
Part One - Pet Stories	1
Laddie and Alex	3
Max and Melissa	13
Alice and Oatmeal Cookies	29
Maggie and Ruth	37
Buck and Leon	45
Shagnasty and Rich	51
Toby and Mrs. Wilson	63
Monte and Bruce	69
Sparks and Jeff	75
Pearl and Marge	87
Juno and James	95
Sadie and Shane	107
Part Two - Vet Stories	125
Pets and Children	127
A Vet and His Pets	133
Shilo	134
Bailee	141
The Dance	149
Timeless Togetherness	155
Aging Together	159
Saying Goodbye	170
A Pet's Final Gift	178
If Pets Could Write	185
Reply	187

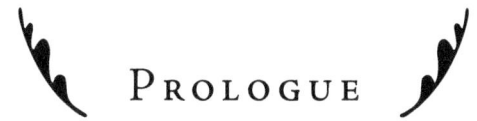

Prologue

"Love is deepest when it hurts the most."

These words from a dear friend – when I was scheduling my old lab, Shilo, for a very serious surgery – reminded me yet again of the power of the mysterious bond between people and their pets.

I had experienced this bond with my own pets and witnessed its melding of joy and suffering in the lives of the many clients I served through 35 years of caring for their pets as a veterinarian. Yet I still needed reminding of the bond's power – and of the mysterious way that the depth of our sorrow over losing a pet is tightly connected with the lifetime of joy provided by our relationship with our pets.

As any devoted animal guardian will tell you, we humans have been uniquely blessed with the ability to attach ourselves to other living creatures. I have come to believe that this attachment has the potential to bring out the very best in our species: our capacity to unselfishly nurture another living creature, whether human or animal. The animals we adopt, protect and love return in kind this capacity to bond. It creates a unique phenomenon of shared nurturing between humans and animals.

My enduring fascination with – and experience of – this bond and the richness it brings to life, led me to want to share what I have learned through it as a guardian and a veterinarian caring for small animals. (Although I have every respect for large animals and their vets, I was a small animal vet from the very start by temperament and training). The best way to convey that richness seemed to be through stories of my own as a vet and guardian—and those of my clients as guardians.

"After nourishment, shelter and companionship, stories are the thing we need most in the world." This quote from author Philip Pullman, best known for the "His Dark Materials" trilogy, nicely sums up the importance I place on storytelling in how we remember and celebrate our pets, and how they help us grieve their passing.

Some of these stories hinge on the unique qualities of pets that make it easier and safer for people to bond with them. These natural traits that build trust between humans and animals make pets what I call natural helpers. Trust is central to our pets enjoying and earning the status of being important family members. Trust is the bond that enables them to frequently take on the role of natural helper during the stormy times that all families must weather.

The living bond between a pet and a person sometimes becomes the sole (soul) source for a person's experience of bonding in life. This bonding is especially miraculous in circumstances where one's ability to bond with another person has been damaged. It's as if this human-animal connection has a life unto itself whose purpose is to seek out union in situations where bonding between humans has failed. The stories of how these natural helpers have literally saved lives are sources of perennial inspiration for me.

Spoiler alert: this book is top heavy with stories about

dogs and their guardians. It's not because cats, or horses, or rabbits, or birds or (insert your favorite pet species here) are any less gifted as natural helpers. Or that they are less accomplished as instructors of living fully in the moment, or that they are not as effective teachers, wordlessly conveying what it means to be fully present for another being in life and death.

The reason dogs feature prominently is that my primary animal bond has been with them, and perhaps that a higher percentage of American households have dogs than have cats. My earliest memories always included a family pet, and my life was the better for having loved those pets. I experienced the presence of this magical bond with pets throughout my boyhood. This certainly influenced me to choose veterinary medicine (with a "small animal" focus) as my life's vocation. The human-animal bond had silently taken root inside of me from the start.

I knew well the joyous side of the bond with my pets, but the other side – the side that causes the pain – was troubling. I can remember times when death visited our home. My grandfather was the first human to leave me, followed by Spook, our regal orange cat, and then by Lassie, a black Lab. All died before I was old enough to think seriously about death.

I later realized that my family didn't talk about death, nor do we as a society. And it was the silence that made death so foreboding. It seemed to my young mind that this silence was a sign that death held a scary secret, a cloak to obscure my ability to see. It was a spark kindling my imagination to conjure up sinister thoughts to fill the unknown.

My early experiences with death went underground during the youthful excitement of my teenage years and continued to be buried under the busy life of a college student competing for a place in the veterinary college. Even as my long, rigorous professional training equipped me with the knowledge, skills and tools to enrich and extend animals' lives, it did not provide the understanding and emotional wherewithal to deal with pet loss. Death equaled failure.

Professors at university could teach me medical science, but people and their pets became my teachers in the art of experiencing and learning through love and loss. The pets took over where school left off. They would, of course, bring suffering, and I would be confronted with the reality of death and grief. I would also experience the wonder of unexpected survival, with its attending feeling of awe over what I called the life force. And the recognition that the two opposing extremes – deep sorrow and great joy – came from a single source: the human-animal bond. I would discover these two extremes are inseparably linked by this bond, making it impossible to experience joy without also encountering the sorrow of loss. This, for me, became a wonderful mystery that I write about in the stories that follow. It is the bond that gave me real passion for my profession; it is what sustained me throughout my career. I know that without it, the science of practicing medicine would not have been sufficient to carry me through.

But it took the better part of a decade of practice before I started the unfinished work of uncovering what lies beneath the silence surrounding death that makes it so terribly foreboding. That exploration led me to the discovery of the union of my heart to the science of veterinary medicine, to become the vet I always wanted to be, and the recognition that our ability to bond is clear evidence that miracles exist.

All I have to do to determine this is to contemplate the absence of the bond – the thought of life without it would be like a world without color; no brilliant sunrises, sunsets, or rainbows; no green of spring nor variegated colors of fall. Only gray. Life itself is not the miracle – the miracle is life infused with the richly colored emotions that only a bond is capable of rendering. And it is truly remarkable that this miracle is further enriched by an entirely different species – the family pet.

When I began writing down the stories for this book, I intended to stay on the "living" side of the bond. Why write about pet loss when it's so dark and uncomfortable that we don't like to be reminded of it. But it would be dishonest and incomplete to ignore the death of the animals with whom we have established deep bonds.

To exclude that suffering would be like writing about the seasons but leaving out winter. And death is similar to winter. Just as spring and summer would lose much of their beauty without winter's cold and darkness, death gives life meaning. And stories soften the acute pain of loss with joyful remembrance of the time we spent with our beloved pets.

If my stories achieve nothing more than helping guardians grieve the loss of their pet and celebrating fully the love, learning and joy the bond has brought into their lives, I will be the happiest vet alive.

Robert Slack, DVM

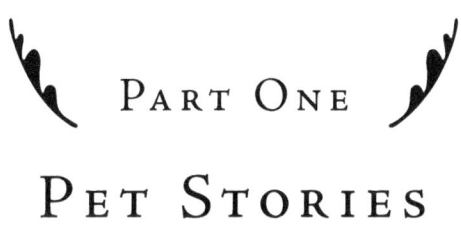

Part One
Pet Stories

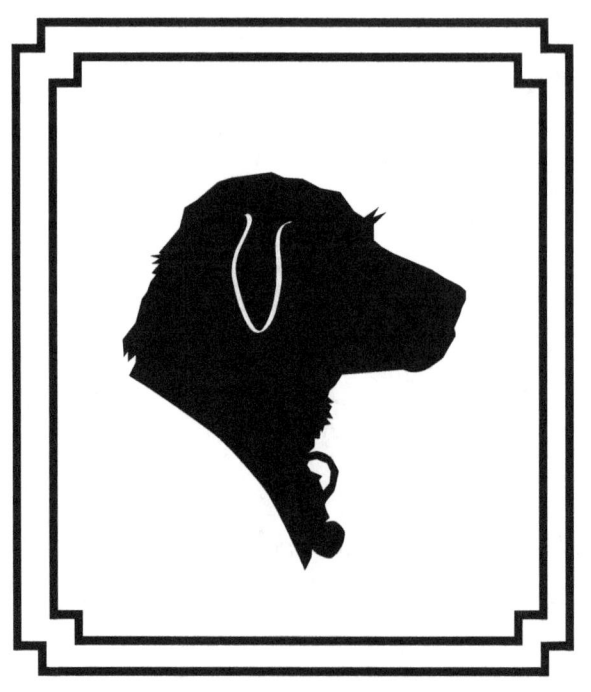

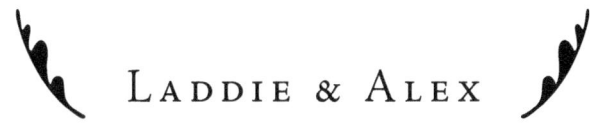

Laddie & Alex

"Good morning," I said, trying my best to sound confident and professional for my very first veterinary consultation in Australia (or anywhere for that matter).

"You're a bloody Yank. Well bugger all!" blurted the elderly man standing across the examination table, a black Labrador retriever sitting by his side. The man stared intently at me in silence, uncomfortably so for me.

Stunned by his abruptness and his obvious displeasure, I stared at the floor trying to gather my wits. He broke the silence: "Me mate's bloody crook, been off 'is tucker for a fortnight, and I biled him out yesterday. Did no good." He again fell silent, his stare hardening. I glanced down at the medical records in my hand and noted my intimidating client's name: Alex.

I had wanted a softer, gentler initiation to veterinary practice, but this was obviously not going to be it. Thoughts tumbled through my head. This elderly man doesn't like Yanks. I have no clue what he meant by crook, tucker and biled. And how does he know I'm a Yank? I had not yet discovered that I had an accent, or that saying "Good morning" instead of "G'day" was a dead giveaway that I was no Aussie.

It was my own curious, restless nature and thirst for adventure that had gotten me to Australia fresh out of vet school at Washington State University. The sunburned continent's unique animal life and the mystery of the Aboriginal dreamtime spoke to me across the ocean, beckoning me to explore a new world.

And now I was certainly doing that as I struggled to understand what my very first client was saying. It might have been comical had not his mate been "bloody crook." As I began examining his mate, I started piecing together what the strange new words meant.

The black Labrador retriever sitting by Alex was named Laddie. The medical chart listed her at 13 years of age, which technically made her a senior citizen. Her grizzled appearance confirmed her advanced years. Graying hair about her muzzle and nearly white circles around her eyes gave her an almost comical owlish appearance, and her frail body seemed to be tacked together with sinew rather than muscle. Her pendulous, seemingly over-full belly stood out in contrast to her otherwise gaunt appearance, and I wondered if her distended abdomen was the product of too much tucker (food) from an indulgent owner or something more serious. I feared the latter.

As I reached out to pat her, I said her name, "Hi, Laddie." She instantly began wagging her tail in a return greeting as she struggled to rise, then apparently thought better of standing and slid back down against her guardian's leg. Few people used the word "guardian" back in the '70s; it would have been "owner" or "master." As my understanding of the nature of the bond between humans and animals has evolved, so too has my language.

Laddie kept wagging her tail vigorously, as Labs are wont to do. Tail wagging is one of a dog's most endearing traits. To me it says, "I don't know you, but I think you're terrific!"

A dog's tail wag is without guile; it offers pure, unadulterated acceptance that blows a human handshake out of the water.

Her tail thumping instantly won me over. I mused how alike Laddie and Alex were. Both were frail and gray, worn with age, and with sagging bellies.

I later learned that my first impression of Alex, like so many of my first impressions as a young and inexperienced vet, was incorrect. He was actually fond of Yanks. Having fought alongside American soldiers defending Australia in World War II, Alex knew them to be courageous and companionable. His initial abrupt demeanor reflected nothing more than Alex's anxiety over Laddie's health.

Alex confessed that Laddie's health had been declining very quickly over the last two weeks. The fortnight. She was very sick. Bloody crook. At first he thought it was just "the arthoritis." As Laddie grew more listless, Alex became more concerned. Finally, when she refused food – tucker – he became alarmed and administered a folk remedy that caused poor Laddie to upchuck. Biled her out. Alex had hoped this would clean out her system and bring back her appetite. No luck there.

Laddie's appetite had always been a very reliable barometer of her health, so her continued refusal was the last straw. Alex brought her into my clinic.

I examined Laddie and questioned Alex about her history before I asked him if I could keep her in the hospital and run some tests. He was reluctant at first, but as he sadly gazed at Laddie, who was now lying quietly next to him, head resting between her extended paws on the hard tile floor, he gave in. "Righty-o, doc, but just for the day," he said.

My relationship with Laddie was to be brief. I ran some blood and urine tests on her, and the results were ominous and conclusive: Laddie was in a late stage of kidney failure. I called Alex and told him to come in so that I could review the results with him. He arrived in short order, and I carefully explained the nature of Laddie's condition. The trembling in his hands increased as he listened, and his voice shook when he asked, "But she'll be right, won't she, doc?" I knew he understood my words, but his heart could not yet accept their meaning.

"Alex", I said, "we could try giving her some fluids – it won't cure her, mind you, but it might make her feel a bit better, maybe buy her a little time." I emphasized "little." He paused before giving his nod for me to try. I administered fluids through an IV and monitored her urine production throughout the day to avoid overloading her system.

The next morning, Laddie began vomiting, her breathing became erratic, and she could no longer raise her head from the blanket that Alex had left for her. "She knows me smell," he'd said as he left the blanket behind. Alarmed by Laddie's rapid decline, I called Alex to let him know that Laddie's health had continued to decline; I told him to come right away.

Laddie died that day in Alex's arms. She stiffened, her chest heaved, and then she laid still, her head resting in the crook of his arm. He sat for quite some time, quietly rocking his friend, his head bent low to hide the tears streaming down his face, dripping onto Laddie's neck. Finally, gently, his head lowered until it rested against Laddie's quiet body.

I watched Laddie's guardian as he left, bent further under the weight of grief, unsteady, with tears in his eyes, without his mate in tow. From a window I watched him climb slowly into his car and rest his head against the steering wheel. His shoulders began to shake uncontrollably as he let his sorrow go in the privacy of his car. After a time, his shaking subsided; he straightened up and sat motionless for some time before starting the engine and driving away.

I later learned that he would arrive at an empty home. His wife had recently died, and Laddie was his sole friend and companion – the only one who had been there to help him fight off the loneliness of his silent house.

As his car disappeared around the corner, a sudden pang of guilt overcame me. The thought that I failed them both played over and over in my mind. Was this a harbinger of things to come? I couldn't escape feeling that I was responsible for this sad outcome. Had I made a mistake? Maybe the blood work was somehow mixed up with that of another pet, and Laddie's condition could have been treated more effectively. My own sadness over Laddie's death and Alex's loss weighed heavily, dragging me down to a very dark place.

In a strange way I felt betrayed. How could I have spent years of training to become a veterinarian only to be left so adrift when faced with what would prove to be so commonplace? I needed to blame someone for causing my bitterness, for my inability to have been more helpful to Alex, to Laddie, to myself. I was unaware that I was grieving.

I had arrived in Australia believing in myself, in my abilities as a veterinarian. My diploma backed me up – it even included the information that I'd graduated magna cum laude – to attest to my qualifications. Yet here I was, foundering, believing I had somehow missed a critical area of my training.

When did my professors warn me that not all diseases

are treatable, that sometimes folks will suffer greatly over loss, that sometimes I would feel deeply the heavy burden of failure. Had no one noticed my innocent faith, my youthful naiveté? I wondered if this was unique to me or if there were others in my profession who struggled with this same sense of helplessness. I was struck by the thought that perhaps I had chosen the wrong profession.

Deep down, I knew I had the knowledge and skills to practice medicine. But now I was faced with the realization that there was this other part of medicine for which I was ill prepared, a part, I would later learn, that could not have been taught. It had to be experienced.

The months following Laddie's death were difficult. The image of the frail old dog resting in the crook of Alex's arm, and his devastation over the loss of his best friend had shaken my confidence. And this was followed by a steady stream of pets with complicated medical problems.

It seemed as if the pets I saw during those first few months in practice were either plagued with obscure syndromes that were difficult to diagnose and equally difficult to treat successfully, or that they'd contracted maladies that were easy to diagnose but unresponsive to treatment – diseases much like Laddie's.

I began to wonder what happened to all the easy stuff I learned about in my medical textbooks, things that were simple to treat and that would let me send pets home happy and healthy.

In the midst of my time in the doldrums, I received my first experience of the power of the human-animal bond to heal a wounded heart. So many times over the years I have heard clients who had just lost a pet say, "Dr. Bob, I can't bear to adopt another pet. It's just too painful to lose them." And then, sooner or later, I would hear an equally common refrain. "Doc, I just couldn't bear to live without a pet. I know I told you I'd never get another one, but…." And I would be presented with a new life – a puppy or kitten, or sometimes an older pet adopted from the local Humane Society. Seeing these older animals adopted was especially gratifying, because I knew it spared their lives. But all of the adoptions buoyed my spirits.

The animal lovers had once again succumbed to the call to care for another creature. They once again entered into that bond, knowing that a season of suffering would follow. But for now, the room would be warmed by their smiles as they watch me check out their newest family members.

Since Alex was the one who brought me my first brush with the part of the bond that brings deep pain, it seems only fitting that it would be Alex who brought me my first experience with renewal: the living bond, that part of the connection that brings joy back into a human's life. Several months after Laddie's death, Alex brought me a small bundle containing a wee black Labrador retriever held in arms that were no longer trembling.

It was a bright sunny morning to go along with Alex's cheery "G-day mate!" as he presented me with a gift of new life. He called his new friend "Li'l Bloke," and I anointed Bloke with his first puppy vaccination. Alex had given in to the call to care for another pet. Once again, he risked the pain of sadness and loss to enter into the bond that gave his life companionship and meaning.

Alex became my first Aussie friend, and he told me about his late wife, his war experiences, and about the land down under. But more than that, he, and his beloved Laddie, introduced me to the sanctity of the human-animal bond.

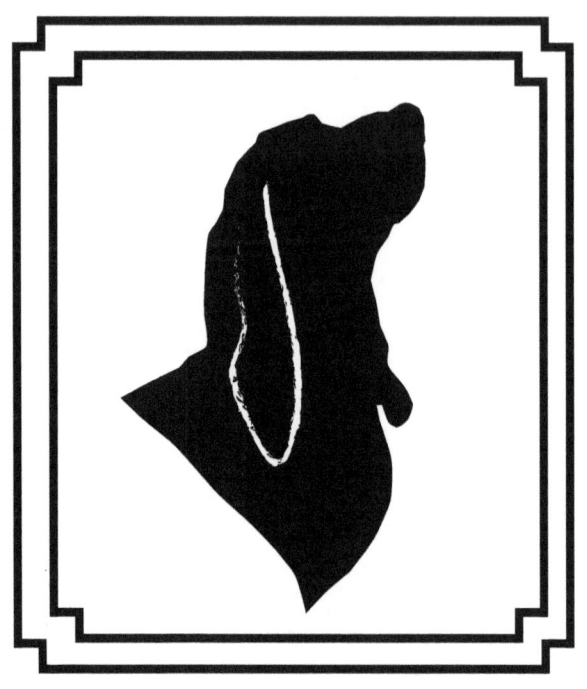

Max & Melissa

I had just entered the treatment area of the hospital when Helen, my receptionist, suddenly ushered in a man with a little girl of seven or eight. His arms cradled a small burlap sack with a large brown ear hung limply out of a slit at one end. The man's eyes moved nervously from me to the girl standing at his side and then back again to me. His drawn face revealed a man desperate to be unburdened of what he held in his arms.

The girl leaned against his side, her arm wrapped tightly about his leg. Her tears had washed down her face leaving tiny serpentine streams, white against the muddy banks of her cheeks. Her fragile chin quivered as she asked in a small, shaky voice, "Please save me little doggie, please." The father nodded as he carefully handed the small burlap bundle over to me, saying, "Please, just try. It was a car that done it."

No further words were needed. The fear in their eyes, the tracks of her tears and the desperate pleading for me to help left me no choice but to utter, "Yes, I'll try." I'm sure my voice must have sounded hesitant, since I really had no idea just what I would find inside the coarse bundle being handed to me.

Helen ushered the man and the girl out into the waiting area. Just as they turned the corner, the little girl glanced back and I caught a faint smile appearing on her face that vanished as quickly as it had arisen. The fleeting smile that carried this child's hope would follow me through the remainder of the day.

As I placed the small bundle on the treatment table, a fold in the burlap fell away, leaving the puppy's head exposed. I instantly recognized that the oversized ear could belong only to a Bassett hound. The pup laid so still, almost lifeless, that there was only the slightest foothold for hope. I could hear the little girl's small voice, a mere whisper in my mind, pleading for me to save her puppy, triggering my memory of Laddie's fate and of Alex's hopes turned to grief. A sliver of fear had wedged itself in my mind, a harsh reminder of the difficult beginning of my work as a veterinarian just a few months before.

I looked more closely at the puppy's head. A dark blue tongue hung listless out the side of its mouth. The pupils were dilated, making the eyes appear coal black and chillingly empty. I quickly slipped my hand along its chest to feel over the heart area. No heartbeat.

The little girl's thin smile again flashed across my mind, reminding me of my promise to try to save the pup. Now the full weight of that promise was starting to press down on me. I felt caught between two warring emotions: the guilt I would feel if I quit now, dashing the hopes of a child, and the fear of failure if I tried and failed. I could hear two voices whispering. The hopeful one said, "Please save me little doggie." The hopeless one said, "This wee pup is far too gone, so you had better quit now!"

I felt immobilized. Both alternatives seemed dreadful. Would it be reckless of me to proceed if I truly believed this puppy was beyond help? Or if I chose to quit, would I deprive this pup of the chance at life?

In the midst of this turmoil a moment of clarity suddenly

came to me. I realized I could not let myself be driven by emotion, allowing it to dictate my decision-making and overpower the discipline of my medical training. If I were to be of any help to any of them, I needed to let the pup's responses to my actions be my guide. I decided to proceed.

Thinking about that day years later, I realized that I wasn't as objective as I had believed. Maybe I had let a little girl's tears influence my judgment; maybe I was a little reckless (that comes with inexperience). But perhaps I just wanted to give this pup a chance at a life he had just barely begun.

I unwrapped Max (whose name I learned only later) from the rest of the dirty burlap bag. I was not prepared for what I uncovered. Max's abdomen had been ruptured like a ripe melon dropped to the floor. His intestines, splayed outside his body cavity, were covered in dirt, gravel, and grass. His pelvis was separated, exposing his large bowel and a ruptured urinary bladder. His tiny scrotum and penis were intact.

The hopeless voice whispered: "Give up now. Isn't it the humane thing to do, to quit? Wouldn't it be easier to give up now and let them know nothing can be done?" I pushed that voice aside.

I was fortunate to have Joanne, a veterinary technician (not the title they had back in the '70s) working with me that afternoon. She was amazingly capable of doing what I would need of her.

I first had to intubate the puppy. I gently slid a tube into his mouth, between the vocal folds and into the windpipe. I now had a direct passageway to administer oxygen. Jo connected this tube to another line that led to a bag hanging from the side of the anesthetic machine, which she quickly filled with oxygen. By compressing the bag, she could inflate Max's tiny lungs with oxygen.

"Okay, squeeze the bag. That's it!" I shouted as I watched his tiny chest expand. "Not too hard; that's it, good."

I began to compress Max's heart. His tiny chest was v-shaped, and his ribs were still mostly soft cartilage, making it easy to massage his heart. I held it in my hand, feeling it trapped between by thumb and fingers.

I compressed the heart several times and then told Joanne to inflate the lungs with more oxygen. She did this several times without success, but still there was no heartbeat. I estimated that less than five minutes had elapsed since the man and the little girl had first arrived.

I asked Jo to get the epinephrine (adrenalin) from the emergency kit. Immediately, she handed it to me, preloaded in a syringe attached to a long thin needle. I quickly slipped the needle between the pup's ribs and directly into his heart. Blood mushroomed back into the syringe, confirming that it was within the heart chamber. I pressed down on the plunger, pumping the stimulant into his heart, removed the needle and continued massaging his heart. Suddenly, I felt a very strong beat. That single beat stood alone, solitary and fearless, against all odds. I felt an answering beat of hope stir within me.

"Jo, give another breath," I urged. There it was – another beat, a pulse from deep within this still body. It sounded a knell that this tiny motionless pup was stirring, pushing back against the enveloping darkness of death. And then came another beat. And another. They continued, very irregular but growing in strength and frequency. "I can't believe this heart," I said. "It's determined to live." I could see Jo was also excited as she watched the puppy wide-eyed. The battle between life and death had begun. It began as that single beautiful beat from a resilient heart, a desperate plea for help.

In critical situations it has always helped me to think of my actions as if I were going into battle. I think it is a way to detach from emotions, quieting the unhelpful voices vying for attention, allowing me to think more clearly, more objectively.

I knew some things about my side of the battle line. I had a known arsenal: Jo's skills, a room filled with medical equipment, my training, and a youthful heart refusing to quit. Max's heartbeat was my first clear sign to continue the fight. Also perched way out on the edge of my mind stood a little girl overlooking the battlefield, her smile a banner of hope, waving as a sign for me not to give in too soon. I felt a wave of confidence creating the calmness I would need, a stillness that allowed me to focus my yet-untested training on the small, fragile creature before me.

A stream of thoughts flowed through my mind. Death, too, had its arsenal: shock, hypothermia, pain, infection, trauma, hemorrhage, possible brain injury, possible fractured spine: all these possibilities were vying for my attention. I was also aware that at the very edge of our battlefield there stalked an unknown. Death does not always reveal all its weapons openly, and I knew I must be vigilant to its wily nature. But it was not death's arsenal that stood out in my mental battlefield. It was Max's heartbeat striking the first blow for life.

"Jo, we've got to get fluids started," I said. Max's heart was producing enough blood pressure that we might be able to get an IV started. Jo was especially skilled at getting a catheter into an incredibly small, partially collapsed vein. She did not disappoint, hitting an almost invisible vein in the puppy's front leg on the first try and connecting it to a line leading to a bag of lactated ringers, a solution of water and minerals that Max needed to fight off shock.

Shock would collapse his blood pressure, which was crucial to keep blood circulating to all his vital tissues, especially his heart and brain. I did a quick search for hemorrhages and was surprised to find very little evidence of bleeding. But as the little dog's blood pressure rose, that could still become a problem.

I shined a light at his pupils, which responded weakly. They did contract, even if not as quickly as normal. I was worried that even if Max survived his uphill battle to live, there was still a very good chance his heart had stopped beating long enough to cause brain damage.

It isn't a great achievement to save a pet only to find him blind or demented from oxygen deprivation. There was no way for me to know the status of his brain function early on, and all I could do was hope that his heart had stopped just moments before I first saw him. That, along with the oxygen now flowing into his lungs and filling his red blood cells with its life-giving energy, was the best chance for minimal brain damage. His youth was on our side.

We moved Max over to the sink area, opened up several bags of saline solution, and began washing away the dirt and gravel from his exposed abdominal organs. Jo used forceps to retrieve the bits of grass and debris not washed away by the solution.

Max already seemed to be improving. His tongue was now completely pink, but he still didn't move at all. Eyelids, tongue, legs, all were completely still. I wondered if Max might have a broken back. Great, I thought, blind and paralyzed.

Pushing away that thought, I was pleased at how quickly we were able to remove most of the debris from his intestines, but I also knew that unseen myriad bacteria must be contaminating his entire abdomen. Antibiotics would be my best hope in dealing with these invisible enemies. I gently placed Max's intestines back into his tiny body cavity and closed the gaping wound with several clamps before transporting him into the surgery room.

The pup's tiny frame seemed even smaller as he lay there on a surgery table large enough to accommodate a Great Dane. The massive surgery light hanging from the ceiling further accented his smallness. It cast a cold brightness upon Max's fragile body, giving him the appearance of a corpse. I fought against that stubborn voice in my head that told me how stupid I was even to consider trying to save this wee mote of an animal. How arrogant! I thought. Was I being cruel to continue?

I was worried about Max's body temperature. Hypothermia was definitely a reliable tool in the enemy camp. I wished we had a heated pad to place him on, but a folded towel to insulate his body from the cold steel of the surgery table would have to do for now. There were still so many variables and so few certainties deciding the fate of the little Bassett.

I looked over at Jo and said, "Stop bagging the oxygen." I wanted to see if Max would breathe on his own. We stood in the quiet of the room staring at his chest. His tongue was still pink from the oxygen we had been artificially administering, and time crawled by as we waited for his system to recognize the drop in oxygen and the buildup of carbon dioxide. It was the increase of the CO_2 that would stimulate his respiration. His tongue began to darken, and I was just about to tell Jo to bag him again. But just there, just then, his chest moved almost imperceptibly. I thought it might be my imagination. Then, there it was, no doubt about it, his first real deep breath taken on his own. I gasped, and realized that I had been holding my own breath while waiting for Max to breathe.

Something new was happening, I was beginning to grow attached to this little guy. My motivation was no longer the little girl with her anxious father; nor was it my fragile ego not wanting to fail. It was Max. I wanted him to live. It would be so unfair for him to die after making it this far.

We were getting far enough into this fray that I began to believe that perhaps death was weakening and the enemy was losing ground.

I began to notice a slight shift in the battle line. Death was beginning a slow retreat. My thinking and actions were becoming more fluid, less tangled in the uncertainties, more focused on each step at hand. I began to believe in my abilities, in myself.

"Jo, keep the anesthetic turned off until we see any sign that he might be feeling pain," I said. Jo glanced down to confirm that the dial was still set on "0," where it had been all along.

I quickly scrubbed in and threw on a surgery gown. I knew Max was grossly contaminated with a wide assortment of germs that could cause any number of diseases (pathology had been one of my favorite disciplines in vet school), but it still felt good, and necessary, to slip into the sterile gloves.

I stepped up to the surgery table and began the slow process of putting Max back together again. The thought of Humpty Dumpty crossed my mind, another fleeting metaphor for what lay before me. I carefully but quickly explored the abdomen. The liver and spleen were not torn. The vessels and membranes that supplied the intestines were miraculously intact. But the bladder was badly torn. I remembered a lecture about this. The professor said, "Always check the bladder when there is trauma to the abdomen. If a pet is hit when its bladder is full, the bladder could very easily be ruptured."

Well, I didn't have to guess about that one. I had never sutured a bladder closed before. I knew it had to be done carefully and with a suture pattern that would prevent leakage. The rupture was irregular, making it difficult to close, but it pulled together, stitch by stitch.

I felt strangely calm. Despite Laddie's death and the difficult cases that followed, here in this quiet room, my mind was clear and I felt confident. My fingers seemed to move freely as if they had a life of their own. I secured the last suture in the bladder and again looked around the abdomen. I noticed no further damage, no bleeding.

I moved to repair the pelvis that had split open. It wasn't a fracture but a separation along the pubic bone, and I was able to bring the two halves back together holding them in place with several wire sutures. I wondered how much nerve damage had occurred. Glancing at the bladder, I was pleased to see it growing in size as it filled with new urine formed by Max's kidneys. This told me two things: the kidneys still functioned, and my sutures weren't leaking.

During surgery, Jo was watching the puppy's color and breathing. He maintained breathing on his own, and he stayed pink. Our battle flag, in fact, was pink, the magnificent color of life moving forward. Max continued his steady march against the retreating foe.

The only task that remained was to close the large tear in the pup's abdominal wall. The muscle layer was not badly damaged. I was able to close the tear, which was really more a separation than a tear, with a continuous suture pattern that saved precious time. I then began closing the skin in a similar manner. I was getting close to finishing his skin sutures when Max's hind legs moved! I stopped, frozen for a moment, to allow what I had just observed to sink in.

I glanced up at Jo and said, "I think he's feeling pain." I hoped this was a sign that his spine was not seriously damaged. If he was moving his legs because he was actually feeling pain, this was indeed a good sign. I slipped the suture needle into his skin once again. It was the final suture to complete his skin closure, and his legs again moved. Max had gone through an entire surgery on oxygen alone; no anesthesia had been turned on throughout his surgery.

I was finished with the surgery phase of Max's perilous journey. As I stepped back from the surgery table, I had trouble standing up straight. I had been hunched over the table the entire time without realizing it. I would learn later to stand more erect during surgery, but that day I didn't mind feeling like an old man. My eyes burned. I had been concentrating so hard during surgery that I had simply stopped blinking. I was exhausted, but exhilarated knowing that Max was still with us.

My thoughts turned to the little girl who might still be sitting out in the waiting area. I asked Jo to see if the puppy's guardian was still there. "Let him know Max is still with us," I told her. "Don't be overly optimistic, but he needs to know that there is definitely more hope now than there was when he arrived."

I was alone with Max. The room was quiet, and in the stillness I became aware once again of my growing attachment to this stubborn little creature. This pup's tenacious grip on life, his refusal to give up in the face of so many injuries, each one capable of causing death, had given me a profound respect for life's resiliency. I reached out and gently felt the soft velvet of his oversized ear and debated how best to manage the pain my awakening friend would most certainly feel.

Jo came back into the room. "I let them know that Max is still with us," she said. I could tell by the lightness in her voice that she, too, was relieved we did not have to give Max's guardian bad news, at least not yet.

Jo helped me carry Max out into the recovery ward, where an incubator we'd scavenged from a human hospital was waiting. She had wisely remembered to turn it on prior to Max's surgery. She carefully lowered him into the welcoming warmth and gently laid him on a soft bed of blankets, adjusted the drip rate on the IV line that was still taped to his tiny front leg, and carefully lowered the lid.

I admired again Max's stubborn refusal to surrender his life, to yield to death's threatening authority. He was pushing back against all odds, creating a bond between us. I wanted him to live.

I remember so well that moment so many years ago. The

windows to the ward were shaded, and the subdued light seemed to amplify the yellow glow given off by the single incandescent bulb inside the incubator. The glow seemed to capture Max's struggle to live. I sat slumped in a chair facing him, remembering his deathly appearance, mesmerized by the tiny movements of his chest, and wondering and worrying over his tenuous hold on life.

I was spent. The fatigue of that grueling day had descended upon me like a wave collapsing on a shore. Maybe I was not myself in that moment, overcome with fatigue, when a sudden feeling of well-being washed over me.

Seeing Max in his incubator struggling as if in defiance of my vision of him lying in a coffin brought me a feeling of deep respect, almost reverence for whatever Max had within him that was protecting him. I was overcome by the thought that something was at work here that was far beyond my knowing and far beyond my doing and it was keeping Max alive. I thought of it as a life force, two words that explain what I cannot fully comprehend.

Surrendering to it is accepting not knowing, and recognizing my limitations and acknowledging how little I really know. That is humbling.

The feeling that visited me that day was new and unfamiliar. Only much later would I come up with a word that adequately described the feeling. The word was awe. That day with Max would mark the beginning of my relationship with mystery, which moved in to take a place in my practice of medicine.

Early the next morning, Jo found me deep asleep on the couch in the staff room still wrapped in my surgery gown. I remember her shaking me by the shoulders.

"Dr. Slack," she said, urgency in her voice, "come quickly. It's Max."

My mind was caught in that shadowy place, half awake and half asleep, but not so unconscious that I didn't feel a sense of dread now rising in me. "I can't take having him dead after all we have been through," was my single thought. I reluctantly followed her into the treatment room, expecting the worst. But there, across the room, standing on his back legs, front legs pawing on the kennel door, stood Max. As my eyes met this unexpected scene, he gave a shrill bark as he danced back and forth on his hind legs.

Was I dreaming? The scene of him lying in his incubator the night before was inconceivable compared with what I was seeing before me now. But several more of the puppy's lively yips drowned out all doubt. This animated little critter, this stubborn hound was too foolish to understand that he shouldn't be with us at all, or at the very least should be lying quietly in the safety of his incubator. Instead, Max looked ready to take on the world.

Jo laughed as she said, "I renamed him Lazarus! I had to take him out of the incubator, because he was all tangled up in his drip line and madder than hell. He was struggling so much that I was afraid he might hurt himself. He's a cheeky little bugger!"

Only a pain sedative could quiet him down. He would not tolerate a caged life even for the few days we kept him under our watchful eyes. Despite my fears about Death's hidden arsenal, the little guy made a full and uneventful recovery.

I had the pleasure of following Max's progress over the

several years I remained in Australia. "His" little girl's name was Melissa, and over time I got to know her and Max a lot better. Max never did quite grow into his ears, and Melissa's tears were replaced with a most radiant smile, a smile that would stay with me over all my years in the practice of veterinary medicine.

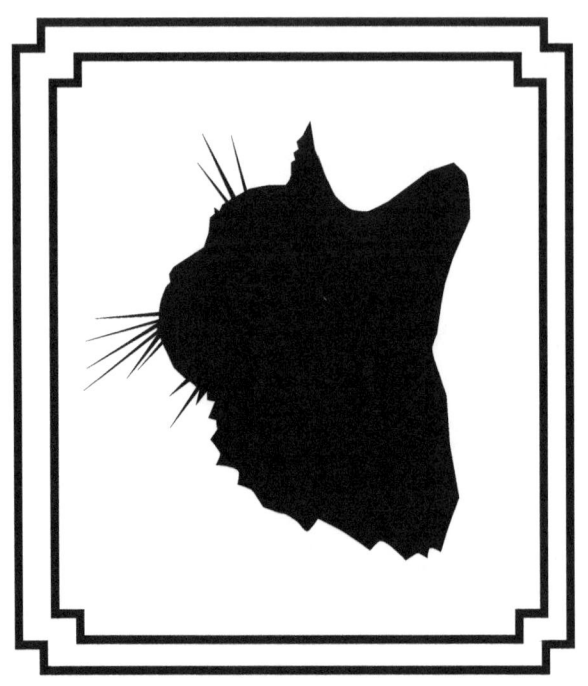

Alice & Oatmeal Cookies

I returned to my home in America after three years in Australia for no other reason than it was time to go. Those years were my initiation into the practice of veterinary medicine.

I am forever indebted to the Australian people for allowing me to practice medicine in their country. Those formative three years were invaluable, giving me the confidence that I had what it takes to be a vet. Since the veterinarian who ran the practice where I worked enjoyed hiring vets from other countries, I had worked alongside colleagues from Australia, New Zealand, Canada, England and Germany. There could not have been a more diverse environment for starting my career. The veterinarians came from different schools of learning and offered a variety of different ways to treat a particular malady. I could then choose which technique worked best for me.

I went home convinced that I could not have chosen a better career to spend my life in. I also came home with indelible memories of many animals and the Aussies who cared for them. Laddie and Alex and Max and Melissa remain foremost among them. They stand as sentinels to remind me to never disrespect the part "life force" plays in this profession or forget that it is the mystery that keeps hubris at bay and keeps me honest with myself.

It brings to mind a lesson I learned from Tom, a Canadian veterinarian that I worked side by side with in Australia. He was by far the most gifted veterinarian I have ever known – and very perceptive. Tom would catch me toying with hubris whenever I got seduced into believing I should be able to unravel every arcane malady that came through the clinic door. When I did, he would laugh, slap me on the back, saying, "Bob, whenever you believe you have all the answers, that's the time when that invisible genie in the sky unzips his fly and urinates on the pillars of science!" To this day, Tom and those two sentinel pets know when to whisper in my ear, warning me whenever hubris begins its seductive dance.

Max was catapulted into my thoughts one afternoon a few years after I had returned to the U.S. My receptionist, Robin, came back to the treatment room carrying a cardboard box. "Dr. Slack, the lady out front is hysterical," she said. "I could hardly understand her but she wants you to look at her cat. She wants to know what she should do. I checked our records, but she's never been in before."

I reached over and lifted the box from Robin's arms and placed in on the examination table and opened the flaps. There, stretched out on her side lay a calico cat (I say her because all calico cats are female). As I peered down at her she lifted her head and immediately two things commanded my attention. I first noticed the look in her eyes as she stared at me. She had what I describe as a pitiful look of complete helplessness, a beseeching look that felt as if she knew I was her last ray of hope.

I felt a pang of sympathy, the same sharp scrape on my heart that I had when I first glimpsed Max after the burlap sack had fallen open. There, protruding from her open mouth was the feathered end of an arrow! She was making pitiful attempts to mew. It was a plaintive sound not quite like I had ever heard before because the arrow was interfering with her ability to make any sound at all.

My eyes quickly went to her chest. She was obviously laboring to breathe. I scanned down her abdomen and could see nothing abnormal until I got to the base of her tail and there, protruding from beneath the tail was the pointed end of that same arrow. It was the pointed tip of a target arrow, not the "V" shape of a hunting arrowhead.

The shocking memory of Max lying on the table with all his overwhelming injuries – and my promise to that little girl that I would try to save him – rocketed back into my awareness. But now, after several years of practice, I was wiser and knew more of the harsh realities of this battle between life and death. Having seen these tragedies – dogs hit by cars, little dogs torn apart by larger dogs – over and over, had had the effect of growing a protective callus around the heart. Here was a seemingly hopeless situation. I had to make a quick decision.

I asked my assistant who was standing next to me to quickly bring Robin back. I needed to talk to her. Robin returned and I turned to her and quickly explained the situation. "Oh, Dr. Slack," said Robin, "this lady has never been in before and she is out there crying. She has no money and if you think nothing can be done she just wants her cat put to sleep."

I looked back into the carrier and again that ancient memory. "This is certainly hopeless, the cat's obviously suffering – do the right thing!" I told myself. I knew euthanasia would end the cat's suffering. I came to a decision even though I knew the chance of saving the cat was slim to none.

"Robin, ask the lady if she would let me try just one thing. I want to make sure this is not completely hopeless. Tell her not to worry about the bill."

I was able to make that offer because I was working with practice partners who respected each other's decisions to care for an animal whose guardian borders on poverty. That is very freeing. Looking back, I don't believe this attitude was abused. At that moment, I knew I needed that kind of freedom.

I cut away the sides of the box so I could get to her without needing to lift her. I placed a tourniquet about her front leg and administered an intravenous anesthetic. I needed her to be motionless and not feeling pain so I could give her one last chance at living. I noticed her body relax as the anesthetic took effect. I grasped the arrow and gently but steadily pulled it back out the direction it had entered. It slid easily, no resistance at all. Once it was out I placed an oxygen mask over her mouth and nose. I then had my assistant start IV fluids. The whole procedure took less than 15 minutes.

My favorite course in vet school was anatomy. We spent many hours in dissection rooms and then reviewed the subject later in surgery and radiology classes. In my mind, I followed the path that arrow took as it traveled through her body all the way to its exit point.

I knew there were so many points along the way where the arrow should have ended her life. It had to have damaged the esophagus or throat area when entering her body. It had then traveled down the neck area reaching the chest. Here it had to have missed the heart and major vessels or else she would have died before making it to the hospital.

When I listened to her chest, I could tell the arrow passed

through the right side. The left side had normal lung sounds, the right side still had lung sounds but they were very moist. That told me that for some charmed reason the lung had not completely collapsed. It was obvious, though, that there was considerable damage.

The next structure the arrow had to penetrate was the diaphragm, the muscular tissue separating the chest cavity from the abdomen. Directly adjacent was the liver; it would be nearly impossible for the arrow not to penetrate this organ and hopefully miss the gall bladder.

From there it became more difficult to know what structures were damaged or missed. The stomach, pancreas, and spleen were all in alignment with the direction the arrow must have taken, but whether it penetrated or slid alongside of these structures I could only guess. Then the coil of small intestines, urinary bladder and large bowel were next in line for the arrow's perilous journey before its exit through the pelvic canal and out the perineal area next to the anus.

My decision was to first remove the arrow and then observe its immediate effect. It might worsen the damage it created in the chest cavity as well as the abdominal area, possibly increasing the risk of hemorrhage. I knew if the digestive tract had been punctured there would be a good chance of contamination of the abdomen. I knew the animal's tenuous grip on life would not survive heroic measures of a surgical intervention so I elected to watch her vital signs and administer supportive care.

So why did I take you down that nasty anatomical journey taken by an arrow? I guess I just wanted to impress upon you that every so often miracles happen. Sometimes pets survive, as Max did, for inexplicable reasons. Call it what you like: luck, serendipity, or a miracle. I like to call it mystery.

Once again I experienced the awesome ability of a living creature's life force to battle against what seems to be insurmountable odds – and survive. And once again I was reminded how little I really know. What did I do? Very little compared to what was going on inside the calico cat's body.

I could boast that I used a technically difficult procedure in pulling an arrow out, as if there were a course in "arrow extraction" that only a select few are able to master. If you believe that, then pigs can fly. But I did do one thing; I decided to give her a chance.

Alice, her name I later learned, went on, as did Max, to make a quick, uneventful recovery. Her vital signs improved, her gums stayed nice and pink, and her breathing stabilized. She neither spiked a fever nor lost her appetite.

Alice earned her release from our hospital after she proved to us she could have a normal bowel movement. Never has a successful bowel movement been met with such jubilation. If cats really have nine lives, I figure Alice used them all up – and then some. Max would be proud of her.

I don't recall the name of the lady who brought Alice to us. She came back many months later. She wanted to pay something for our work but all she could afford was a plate of oatmeal cookies. That was enough for us.

I like to think that maybe Alice and Max met up in another life. They certainly would have mutual disdain over the other's poor choice of species before comparing notes about their narrow escapes from death. They, too, might arrive at the conclusion that more was at work inside them than what could be conjured up in the imperfect mind of a two-legged animal doctor.

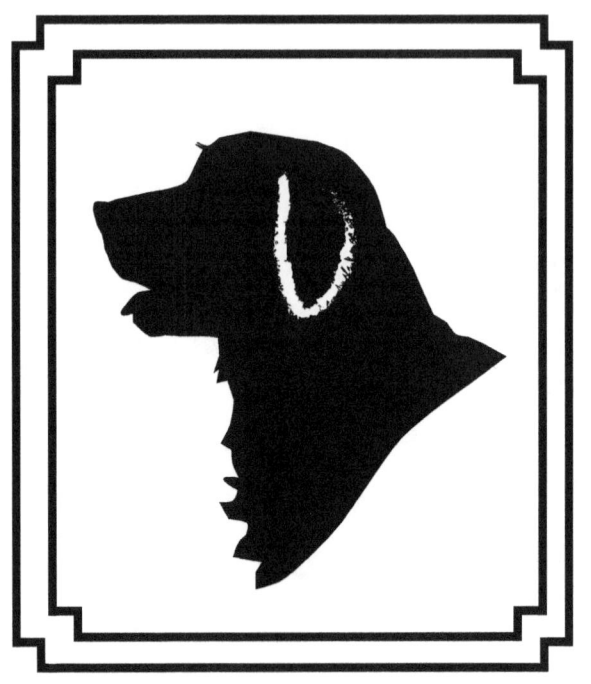

Maggie & Ruth

"I hate to do this to you, but you have an unscheduled appointment. Ruth Hart is here with Maggie. Ruth is crying. I put her in Room 1. I think it might be a euthanasia, Dr. Slack." An unexpected euthanasia is a tough way to end my day.

Maggie is an elderly golden retriever that has been gallantly battling the relentless progression of arthritis, a condition for which there is no cure. I wasn't prepared for this. I knew she was struggling, but perhaps something else has happened. Why couldn't my last consultation of the day be simple: a puppy or kitten in for a health checkup and shots? An appointment that allows both pet and guardian to leave happily.

I have a few moments to review Maggie's medical records before going into Room 1. I note the many repeat prescriptions for arthritic-pain medication dating back several years. I have worked hard at helping Maggie over these years, adjusting medication dosages, adding different ones to the mix, keeping her weight down, instructing Ruth to continue taking her on brief walks to help with her muscle tone. But her arthritis has been a ruthless opponent.

Maggie is 14 now, old for a golden, but sometimes our love for our canine companions and our own sense of time delude us into thinking that time for our particular pet is somehow different. We who love our animals want to stretch time out, to make it last longer.

Entering the room, I'm confronted by Maggie lying on a blanket on the floor. In her mouth she holds her familiar yellow tennis ball. Her head slowly turns toward me, ball clinched firmly in her mouth, eyes fixed on me with what seems to be a defiant stare – a look that seems to say, "Just try to take my ball away!"

The presence of the ball in her mouth has caught me off guard, unexpectedly triggering memories of Maggie in her youth. Through the years, she has always arrived for her yearly exams with her ball held stubbornly in her mouth. This made examining her mouth a bit difficult, as she playfully resisted my attempts to remove the ball.

I learned through the many stories Mrs. Hart would tell that the ball represented what was best in Maggie. She lived to retrieve. Mrs. Hart even purchased one of those slings to help her throw the ball, for her arm tired much more quickly than Maggie's legs did.

The thought of Maggie racing to retrieve the ball brought back memories of Abby, my first Labrador retriever. She was a classic example of her breed and lived a long life before I, too, had to face the painful decision that Ruth now faces. Both Maggie and Abby carry the retriever genes, one golden, the other Lab.

Abby, like Maggie, had her day in the sun when her body was still agile, before time had inexorably stiffened her into old age. Abby used to run with such a fluid grace, a gait more like gliding than running, before she slowly deteriorated and her gait became stilted, the telltale signs that arthritis was upon her. She was only 10 years old. I was amazed that her enthusiasm to take our daily walks into the nearby woods had not diminished. She could tell by how I dressed that it was walk time. She bounced up and down, twirled around, all the while making continual coaxing moves toward the door. Yes, she knew when it was time.

All these memories came flooding back at the sight of that ball clinched in Maggie's jaws, symbolic of two wonderful pets that found their joy in life in retrieving.

I was caught off guard by the unexpected contrast of Maggie's appearance on the floor of the exam room to the stories of her boundless energy. I was thinking of how Maggie's deterioration has paralleled my own pet's aging. A sudden wave of sadness washed through me, exposing my own tendency to deny how quickly time passes for our four-legged companions.

In my mind's eye I still see Maggie as a vibrant retriever in her prime, racing across the grass in pursuit of her ball – a ball thrown as many times as the family's love could manage with the bottomless depth of energy a retriever has for just that: retrieving.

In my mind, she becomes Abby, who relentlessly pestered me to throw the stick, the ball, the Frisbee: anything would do. Just throw it!! Throw it across the field, into the water or into a stand of bushes. How quickly and with what agile grace she pursued her ball, leaping as though gravity were dismissed for the duration of this game. Then, with a sudden scoop at full speed, she would masterfully snatch the ball from its outward-bound path and, in the blink of an eye her direction would change until she was speeding toward me. She would drop the ball, disgusting with drool, at my feet.

And her eyes – so intent, so totally in the moment – would fill with adrenalin-charged excitement that I only wish I could muster for myself. We were playing it: The Game.

The game I thought would never end.

These dogs are born to retrieve, and we humans can only dream of something so simple that could make us so happy. That knowledge, that memory, was the source of my sudden pain. It was the pain of recognition of times gone by, when joints and stamina defied fatigue, when speed and agility were effortless and reliable, when eyes danced with abandon, with excitement for The Game.

The sight of that old tennis ball transforms Maggie in my mind into one of those images of precious youth that belie the stark reality of encroaching age. She suffers under the ravages of time. Her body has been eroded by nature's time, which has deposited her here before me, worn down, her eyes now dull, her coat lusterless and patchy, her wasted muscles making it difficult for her even to stand.

I don't want to be here in this room. I feel what all guardians feel: "How could this moment arrive so soon? I feel the weight of this moment as if my own pet were present. I am feeling sorry for myself and for Abby's death, as well. I remember when it was Abby lying on a blanket on the floor of Room 1.

I bend down to pat Maggie's head and I look up at Ruth, Maggie's loving guardian. Her eyes are swollen, and I can tell she's been fretting about the inevitability of this moment for some time. Her tears filled the lower rims of her eyelids, and when I begin to talk to her they quickly overflow and run down her face. I have known Ruth since Maggie's puppyhood, 14 short years.

"Ruth," I begin, "I knew this time was coming, but somehow it seems unfair that it's arrived."

"Dr. Bob," she replies, "I've been lifting Maggie by putting a towel under her belly to help her, but now I haven't the strength. The distraught woman bursts into tears and sobs. "She's so upset when she soils her blanket."

I wait.

"I hope I haven't waited too long,'" she continues. "Maybe I should have come in sooner. I feel so guilty! But then I think I should give her just one more day. Just one more day."

Her sobbing muffles her words. Then, clearly, I hear, "I know it's time."

I look at her. She seems so fragile, so vulnerable. "Ruth, arthritis is difficult. It is a fading kind of disease that keeps us guessing about when it's time. You have been a faithful caretaker throughout Maggie's life, especially over these last few years. I think you know that."

She nods. A smile flickers across Ruth's face, a fleeting moment of reprieve from her anguish.

I continue, "Ruth, the bond you have with Maggie has always been so obvious to me. And I'm not just talking about your attachment to Maggie that is so clearly present every time you come to see me, but also her attachment to you. I believe it is that very attachment that brings you here now; love is behind your decision to end her life. I have great admiration for the courage it takes to not allow Maggie to suffer beyond what your heart knows is right."

As I talk, I notice Ruth nods as I mentioned the part about her heart. She sobs, "Yes, I have struggled dearly over that very thing. I decided I would not let guilt win over this morning and keep me home, make me cancel my appointment with you. And you're right, I truly believe my love for Maggie is what brings me here."

Hearing this I have a quiet inward sigh of relief. I know guilt has lost its power to undermine Ruth's resolve to be Maggie's guardian. She is free to intervene in her beloved animal's unnecessary suffering.

Ruth's sigh is long and deep. "I know I am doing the right thing," she says. "It's just so hard."

This is not the time to encourage her to try another medication. We have already been down that path. I know it's time. There is no confusion about what is happening.

Ruth kneels down to stroke Maggie's shaggy hair. Maggie holds her head up and stares quietly into Ruth's eyes, the ball firmly in place. She embraces Maggie, holding her, head against head. I feel my throat tighten. I clip a tuft of hair that obscures a vein on her hind leg and gently place a tourniquet to make it plainly visible. I have prepared Ruth for what will happen, explaining that it will be just like administering an anesthetic for a surgery, only this time the medicine is stronger and death will be quick and painless.

I begin administering the solution. I can see Maggie starting to relax. That's when the ball falls from her mouth. Then something happens that I shall never forget. Maggie seems to overcome the forces of death for just an instant. She suddenly breaks loose from Ruth's embrace and snaps up that yellow ball with such speed and determination that both Ruth and I are amazed.

It's as if she didn't want to enter death without it. And she didn't. The moment the ball was re-secured in her mouth, she passed on. I looked up at Ruth and nodded. No words passed between us, but we both knew what the other was thinking: we had just witnessed the indomitable spirit of a natural retriever.

The ball would remain in Maggie's mouth. We felt it would be wrong to take it from her. And so Maggie was cremated with the ball still firmly grasped between her teeth, a retriever unto death.

It is always humbling for me to witness the courage of folks like Ruth who, against the strong pull from their hearts to hold on, are able to let go. It is a pure act of unselfishness that must come from a very good place deep within the soul, a place that is able to transact what might be called the great exchange: the taking away of suffering from a pet and taking on that burden for oneself. Can there be any higher example of what is good in our humanness? I am truly humbled by such acts of courage.

And I was uplifted to know that guilt had failed in its attempt to claim a place within the sanctity of Ruth's grieving, her place of such deep surrender.

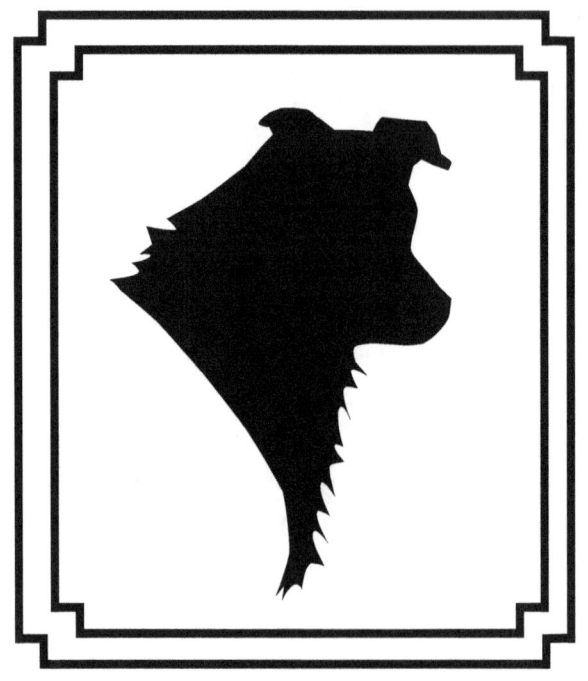

Buck & Leon

"He has cancer."
"What did you say? says Leon. "I can't hear too good."
"Buck has cancer," I repeat, raising my voice.
Silence.
"Cancer, you say."

Leon looks down at Buck, his 12-year-old Border collie. Leon's eyes begin to moisten. Buck must sense the change in his guardian. Is it Leon's sadness – or fear – that brings Buck's ears suddenly erect, eyes sharply attentive, as he stares up at Leon?

He is a big man, a farmer, with large, thick hands. His leathery face has been honed by wind and sun from long summers spent in a tractor's seat. He is one of a dying breed: men who work the soil of their small, endangered farms, resisting the appetites of larger farms that devour those in their way.

"He has cancer, and that's why he's so tired, why he is breathing that way." Buck was in several weeks before, and the tests I ran confirmed my worse suspicions that the source of his labored breathing was a cancer – a very aggressive and evil kind of cancer – that had spread throughout most of his lung tissue.

Buck is more than just a working dog whose job is to run coyotes off or sound an alarm at strange sounds in the night. He has been Leon's sole companion since Leon's wife passed on a year before. He is his master's faithful friend, his partner in labor. Every summer, all summer long, Buck has trailed alongside Leon's tractor, down those long furrows, row upon row. Leon and Buck have been inseparable from sunrise to nightfall as though the soil had grown them together. Buck was as much a part of Leon as the faded coveralls he wore.

"I don't think Buck has a lot of time left," I say, quietly. Leon is the kind of man who can handle my bluntness, but as his eyes settle on mine I feel such sadness that I have to look away. The shared weight of our knowing has forged a heavy bond between us.

"How will I know when it's time?" Leon's voice is stolid, flattened by the toughness wrought from years of wondering when rain might come to break a drought. His outward toughness is betrayed by the tears trailing down his tanned cheeks.

"I think you will know." My reply is honest. "Watch his breathing. When he works too hard at it, you let me know."

"I can do that," he says.

"Take him home, Leon. Take him someplace he knows, a place he enjoys. I don't think it will be too much longer."

Silence again hangs over us. "You have a hard job, Doc."

I'm caught off guard, startled by his concern for me. I am humbled by these unexpected moments when words penetrate my doctor role and strike to the heart of why I chose this profession.

"I think I'll take him down by the pond. We go there a lot in the summer, after a hot day. It's cool there in the evening. He likes to wade out into the water," Leon laughs. "He never goes out too far though. Doesn't like it when his toes can't feel the bottom."

Such a brief time passes before Leon and Buck are back.

Leon is distraught. He sits looking at me and says, "It's time. I know it's time. It's not right to wait any longer."

Buck is sitting at his side looking only at him, the same steady gaze as before. He isn't doing well, his sides heave as he tries to fill his lungs with air. Yet it seems as though he is more worried for his master than himself, perhaps confused by Leon's grief.

I nod knowing that nothing more needs to be said. I return with a syringe. Tears are flowing. Leon wipes his eyes with a hard, rough hand, then reaches into his coveralls for a hanky and blows his nose. I kneel down beside Buck, and he looks at me for the first time. He's struggling to breathe.

I have been here so many times, next to a suffering pet, feeling the full burden that comes when I know I have so little to offer. The irony is harsh, having to turn from my training to sustain life to ending it. It is always a struggle, this letting go, and yet I accept this responsibility knowing that I must be there to end a pet's suffering. This is what must be done when the time comes.

I am witness to Leon's courage, the courage behind the grief. It is so very hard to act on knowing it is time. Leon's burden is palpable. I must hold fast to my deep conviction that sudden death will triumph over the slow suffering of this insidious disease that gnaws away at those few small remnants of life that Buck still clings to. If we wait any longer, the cancer will gnaw into his dignity.

Unlike an aged wolf, he can't wander off to find a dark hidden place, perhaps a small den beneath an upturned tree, pushed over in a sudden mountain storm – a place to crawl into and wait for death to lead him away. With no root to curl up under, Buck is protected by his guardian, Leon. He trusts that his guardian will make that faithful decision to give him that quiet resting place in a different way, when it is time.

Buck dies quickly and peacefully. Just a deep sigh, and then silence. Leon seems suddenly older as he lowers himself slowly to the floor, joints stiff from a life of labor. Breathing hard, he reaches out until his fingers run through Buck's soft fur for the last time. He then grasps the counter, pulls himself up, and through trembling lips he whispers, "Thanks, Doc. Like you said, I'd know when it was time. It was time."

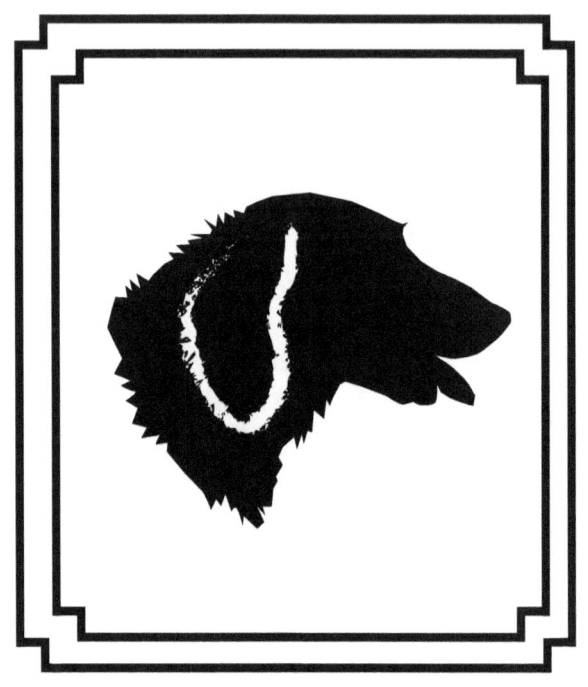

Shagnasty & Rich

About 15 years into my veterinary career, I knew it was time for me to make a change. A big one. I had begun to experience fatigue. Maybe it was normal to have this weariness follow me through my day this many years out of school. But something deeper was calling out for my attention. Something wasn't quite right with me. This was not the kind of fatigue that comes naturally after a hard day's work; this was different, a malaise of a different kind. I was suffering from the very nature of the bond that had stolen itself into my practice of medicine.

That side of the bond that had brought pleasure to my work was succumbing to that other side, the one that brings sorrow. Even though the positive outcomes I experienced with my four-legged patients far outnumbered those that brought sorrow, it was more the sadness that followed me home each evening – that was the haunting heartache I was feeling. I realized that until I came to grips with this grief within myself it would diminish my ability to shepherd heartbroken clients through that tough time when ending their pet's life was at hand. That awareness hastened my decision to leave medicine and pursue a counseling degree. By that time I had been back in the U.S. for 12 years.

I met Rich when I worked as a counselor in a treatment center for addiction. Rich was in his late 20s. He had been in and out of several treatment centers for his alcoholism, and he believed this was his last chance. If he couldn't make it this time, he feared his life would be over. "I don't have another relapse left in me."

Rich had lost all his "normal" friends – or they'd lost him – years ago. When he got drunk he got crazy, and all his friends had drifted away to be replaced by drunks like Rich. "If you only know drunks, where do you go when you leave treatment but back to the only 'friends' you have?" Rich asked.

In one group session, a fellow alcoholic told Rich he needed to find new sober friends, to give Alcoholics Anonymous (AA) a chance. He knew Rich's history of leaving treatment and hanging out in taverns, sipping pop so he could be with his "friends." It was always just a matter of time before beer replaced the soft drink. The streetwise member gave Rich a blunt breakdown. "You know you don't go to a whorehouse for a kiss, and you sure as hell don't go to a tavern for a Pepsi."

Rich wanted sobriety this time. He'd lost the defiant attitude he had carried with him through all his other attempts at getting sober. The street had beaten him up badly, physically as well as emotionally. He wanted to surrender his anger, to give up this life that was heading rapidly downhill. The doctor told him his lab tests indicated that he still had a liver, but that wouldn't last if he continued drinking. He cried the morning after he received the news that his liver had not yet given up on him. He was broken, and his tears were his first outward sign of surrender.

It's difficult for a drunk to admit to being broken. For an alcoholic to surrender means that he has to admit that he has lost control of his life. He makes numerous promises to himself that he won't drink. He makes this promise with good intentions. Rich once stopped drinking for almost a month. He described it as his "dry" drunk, meaning that he was angry and miserable the entire time and that he obsessed continually about wanting to drink. He failed.

Each failure deepened his shame, and he once said in a group session, "I know I've made a lot of mistakes, but now I've come to think of myself as a mistake. I have no real friends. Who could possibly like me? I don't even like myself!" He covered his face with both hands, slumped over until his elbows rested on his knees, oblivious to the attempts of others in the group to reach out to him – to accept him.

I asked Rich into my office, and we talked about life outside of treatment. He had written me a note the previous day, telling me that he wanted to talk. He was a lonely man, and he admitted that the time he spent in taverns helped to soothe his loneliness. I asked if he had any sober friends. "None at all," he answered frankly. We talked about AA and why he didn't attend. He said he felt he didn't belong because he was always too scared to talk, to share the story of his affair with booze. Rich was so burdened with shame that he couldn't bring himself to open up in a group. Even in treatment he kept his story shallow, revealing only a sliver of himself.

I realized Rich was headed for another relapse even before he left our treatment center. His isolation was palpable, and unless he found a way to connect with people, he wouldn't make it. I felt we needed to come up with a plan, something creative to give him a sense of belonging. I felt some hope for Rich because he had finally surrendered the defiant anger that had been his "brand." Being a bad dude was better than being invisible, he told me.

Rich wouldn't look at me during our sessions. He just stared out the window or down at his feet the entire time.

His note asking to see me was a cry for help, a sign that he trusted me enough to be sitting here in front of me, and I felt a glimmer of hope for him.

We needed to find a home for him outside the tavern. His insurance only gave him 30 days in rehab, and this was barely enough time for him to stabilize from the physical effects of withdrawal from his heavy drinking. It certainly didn't allow him time to deal with the chaos found at the bottom of a bottle. Rich would be discharged in less than a week.

I came up with a plan inspired by my experience as a vet and pet guardian and a therapy technique I came upon while taking courses in counseling. The technique developed by Carl Rogers focuses on the qualities that allow a therapist to build trust with his or her clients. I realized that building trust was really about bonding with a client.

Rogers pointed out that there are certain natural qualities a person must have in order to become a successful client-centered therapist: unconditional acceptance (which includes the ability to forgive, listen, and be present), empathy and genuineness.

What caught my attention was the fact that these qualities are not always present in humans in sufficient strength for them to become effective client-centered or Rogerian therapists. I also realized that almost all pets, especially dogs, have these qualities from birth. They are natural helpers.

Pets accept us exactly as we are. That's as simple a definition of unconditional acceptance as I have heard. They don't criticize, and I believe that they wouldn't, even if they could talk. Pets are also able to forgive us without resentment, another sign of unconditional acceptance. They need only the smallest reason to forgive.

Pets are good listeners, too. Quite a few clients admit that they not only talk to their pets, but also swear on a box of pet treats that their pets listen – and even understand. The feeling of being listened to creates a strong bond. Many of us only pretend to listen. Too often we take part of what we hear and summarize what we think the other person is trying to say when he or she just wants to be heard.

Our pets are good at being present, another component of unconditional acceptance. An article I once read gave this wonderful example of this presence.

"I can't think of anything that brings me closer to tears than when my old dog, completely exhausted after a hard day in the field, limps away from her nice spot in front of the fire and comes over to where I'm sitting and puts her head in my lap, a paw over my knee, and closes her eyes, and goes back to sleep. I don't know what I've done to deserve that kind of friend."

Empathy is the second essential quality for gaining trust and forming a bond. Pets can do it without saying a word. Maybe words can even get in the way of empathy. A wagging tail can sometimes express more empathy than comforting words. Dogs are incapable of a fake tail wag – or wiggling in excitement to greet you. I believe their whole being exudes empathy: honest, sincere feeling.

Genuineness, or authenticity, is the third quality. I laugh at this one because all pets are incapable of being anything but real and genuine. That's what I love about them. What you see is what you get. Our pets are incapable of putting on a facade. Has it ever crossed your mind that your pet is just pretending to like you?

This genuineness is communicated without words. It has been estimated that more than 90 percent of communication between humans is non-verbal, conveyed though voice tone, eye contact, gestures, and touch. Sometimes misinterpretation of our words leaves us feeling misunderstood, unaware that our body language is totally out of sync with our intentions. Pets just don't have that problem.

Another characteristic that I have found essential as a therapist for building trust – touch – was not included in Roger's list. One of my respected teachers told me that people need hugs: four a day to survive, eight to maintain, and 12 to grow. Touch is one of the most elemental ways we feel cared for. It's sad when teachers and other caregivers withhold their "hugs" for fear they might be interpreted as inappropriate. My suspicion is that most children fall far short of enough hugs to thrive.

This is where our friends the dog and cat come in. Even though they have no arms, they are the quintessential recipients of hugs. They specialize in welcoming free, safe, abundant, sincere hugs. In their acceptance of our hugs, they convey all the traits of a Rogerian therapist: unconditional acceptance, empathy, and genuineness.

I believe touch to be such an essential part of our bonding with animals that human-animal touch could be used almost interchangeably with human-human touch. Have you ever seen a child hugging a pet and not smiling? It may be that hugs are so powerful in forming a bond because pets need hugs as much as we do. Touch creates a bond because it is mutual in our natures: both people and pets have an innate need to nurture and be nurtured. This is a true gift. Think of your own pet's special ways of making you feel unconditionally accepted and loved.

One year I was invited to be a trainer for a group of high school students selected by their peers to be Natural Helpers. This program started in response to several suicides in our school district. The thought was that maybe troubled students might seek out a peer, a Natural Helper, when they were feeling unsafe or intimidated or too ashamed to talk to a parent or a school counselor. We needed to train these Natural Helpers with communication skills that would help them deal with typical school problems, especially those arising out of bullying. We paid particular attention to training the students to recognize problems of a serious nature. Here, their training was focused on developing referral skills to help them convince the troubled student to seek professional help.

This was the interesting part. I interviewed several of these Natural Helpers to determine why they thought their peers had selected them as people they would seek out if they had a problem. I wasn't surprised to find out that these students displayed the same qualities as pets: acceptance, empathy and genuineness. The answers I got from the Natural Helpers were unpretentious: "They just thought I was easy to talk to." "Maybe they knew I wouldn't judge them or criticize them." "I think they knew I was a good listener." The interesting part was that these Natural Helpers were not the cheerleaders, the jocks, the groupies, or members of any other popular clique. They stood out because of their natural ability to gain trust.

My experience as a guardian, a vet, a counselor and a trainer of Natural Helpers has convinced me that while our pets can't be elevated to the status of therapists, they are indeed our natural helpers. Their natural traits build trust, and establish a bond between us.

Now back to the plan for Rich. My confidence in a pet's ability to help people led me to ask Rich – friendless and in despair if he would consider allowing me to find him a sober friend to be there for him when he was discharged from the treatment center.

He looked at me as if I were crazy. "Get me a friend?" he said, his voice rising. "No way. I can find my own friends." We talked about how he had in the past been unable to develop a normal non-drinking friendship, and he agreed he really had no idea what a friendship really felt like or how to go about finding one. I asked him if he might consider a dog.

His faced dropped. "A dog? Are you kidding me, Doc?" He had begun calling me Doc after hearing about my veterinary history; he knew that I was a great advocate of having canine friends. Once, in a group session, he had reminisced about a dog he'd once had as a kid growing up on his dad's farm. They used to go hiking together in the summer, up in the hills behind the farm. "Those were my best days," he said.

I could hear nostalgia in his voice. I knew he loved animals by the way his voice softened whenever he spoke about his Collie dog, Lacy, and his sadness over losing her to old age while he was still in high school. That's when the idea of bringing a pet back into his life started to make good sense. He would need a friend, especially over the first few months following discharge from our center when he would be most susceptible to relapse.

Several days later, Rich asked to meet with me again. I hoped it was about dogs. I truly thought that a dog might be, at least for the moment, his only chance at staying sober.

"I've been thinking about what you said, Doc, about getting a pet. You know, that might not be a bad idea." I smiled to myself, thinking that just maybe we'd hatched something that could work.

I knew that shame was a huge part of why Rich was having such a struggle in developing friendships. Shame paralyzes. It has the power to send a person into dark places. A pet's ability to unconditionally accept a person was unique to the four-legged world. I believed it just might rub off on Rich and help him on the long road back to accepting himself. But right now we needed to find him a dog friend – and soon.

We spent his last week in treatment figuring how best to go about locating an animal friend before he had to leave. I was a bit worried that if he was unable to remain sober, a pet might suffer the consequences. But I thought it was worth the chance. I knew from our earlier conversations that he would try hard to care for a pet. He certainly had a soft spot in his heart for dogs, and I believed he would take care of one if given the chance. With a little luck, the responsibility of caring for a pet would give him a reason to stay sober.

Then I had to get permission from our administrator to go along with our plan. After listening to my reasons for suggesting this unusual approach to recovery, he agreed, "Bob, I've heard of a lot of crazy 'fixes' to help folks get sober. But in this case, it just might be the right direction to go." I left his office hoping I was not setting Rich up for another failure. But nothing else had worked. I remembered an adage that seemed to fit: "If what you're doing isn't working, do something different."

The next day Rich and I took the clinic van and headed out for the local Humane Society. He spent a long time looking at the motley collection of pets. One kennel after another, down the rows he went. By the time we got to the last kennel in the row, he was sobbing, "Doc, they're just like me. They got no home! I want to make a home for one of them."

His sudden show of emotion was startling. Rich was more animated than I had seen throughout his entire treatment stay.

We came back the next day and he picked out the ugliest critter in the lot: shaggy tangled, yellowish hair, a long body, with stubby, crooked legs. I guessed he must be a cross between a Basset hound and a Golden retriever. He was in the very last kennel, and fastened to the kennel door was a tag with that day's date written in bold red letters.

I looked at Rich, "You sure about this one?" He laughed. "He's not the best looker, but I can tell he really likes me. I haven't felt liked for a long, long time." As we were leaving, I went over to the kennel attendant and asked him about the date posted on the kennel door, and he smiled, saying: "The director has let me keep that mutt around way past the normal time before we'd have to put him down. Everyone here got sorta attached to him. Today would have been his time to be euthanized, but then you folks came around!"

The doubt I had about whether I was doing the right thing, talking Rich into getting a pet vanished. There couldn't have been a clearer sign that this road was the right one.

Rich left treatment with a bag of dog food and his new

friend, Shagnasty. He drove off in his pickup, and I could see Shagnasty's head poking out the side window, mouth wide open and tongue dangling. I swear that pets can smile.

Rich reported to me weekly for a number of months. He always arrived on time and sober and with Shag, as he now called him, in tow. We spent our time together talking about friendships and staying sober.

"You know, Doc, when I take Shag for his walks, kids come running up to me and ask about him. They want to know his name, why his legs are so short, how come he's so ugly. They want to pet him. You know, Doc, he's such a great dog; everyone loves Shag. And I like talking to the kids. I talk to Shag, but it's different than talking to people; they talk back. I figure if people can like my dog, then maybe they could like me, too."

It wasn't long after that that Rich told me he'd given AA another try. "You know," he said, "it isn't that bad. I think I'll get one of those sponsors you've been bugging me about." I do believe the bond Rich had formed with his sober four-legged friend helped him bridge the gap into the human world.

Eventually, I lost track of this young man and his dog. But I was in a group session about a year after my last conversation with Rich, when an older man, who knew I was a vet, said, "Hey Doc, I was at an AA meeting a while back and this guy came in with the strangest lookin' dog I ever seen. Big yellow dog with stubby legs." I smiled. Must have been Shag.

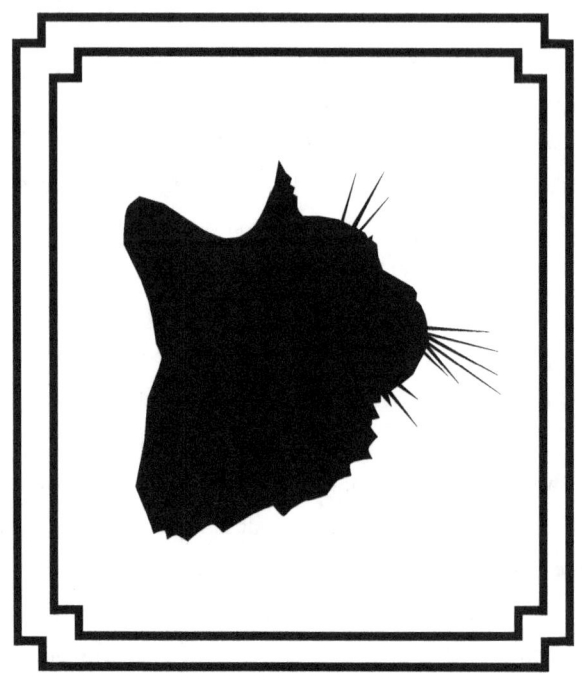

Toby & Mrs. Wilson

After three years of study, a degree in counseling and work experience in that field, I returned to my veterinary practice, refreshed, renewed and with a new appreciation for – and, I hoped, improvement in – communication skills. I combined working with pets with part-time working with people.

Our hospital bestows titles to deserving members of our clinic in recognition of their notable talents. I, for example, was given the infamous title of "Bowel Ranger" in recognition of my surgical skills in removing infected anal glands from anally impaired canines. On the other hand, my partner Vern was dubbed our resident "Micro-man" because his undergraduate training in microbiology had resulted in superior sleuthing skills in finding and destroying bugs–mainly bacteria.

Getting overly attached to a title can sometimes elevate the ego to dangerous heights. When one pokes his puffed-up head through the clouds he is at risk of a mighty fall. The ancient Greeks knew this excessive pride well and made up a name for it: hubris.

Hubris is contagious. I caught a serious case of inflated ego after completing an evening course in "interpersonal communication skills" at a local college. The clinic staff bestowed the title "Master Communicator" on me. With the title came the distasteful task of resolving conflicts, especially those arising from dissatisfied clients. Playing this "role" set me up for a mighty fall, with Mrs. Wilson playing the part of very unhappy client.

Mrs. Wilson had a tender heart for orphaned cats, but

a hardened one for humans, veterinarians included. She had become the neighborhood rescuer of stray cats. Whenever she found one she would quickly bring it to our clinic to have him or her checked out and vaccinated. I would neuter the tomcats and spay the females and she would then become the adoption agency to find them good homes. I have to admit I respected Mrs. Wilson's concern for the abandoned animals; it helped offset the disdain she felt for the two-legged species.

She was not well received by our receptionists because of her condescending attitude and constant complaining about anything that she felt was less than perfect. Mrs. Wilson always arrived dressed to the nines, in high heels, heavily made up, and not a hair out of place. Her outfit gave the impression that she was about to interview for a very important position.

I had no idea how she got along with her husband, but guessed he was a man of considerable patience because she was an unrelenting bully. I spent many meetings with her in the "quiet room" resolving conflict. In retrospect, we should have sent her packing after the first few run-ins.

One sunny afternoon she came barging through the clinic door, a dark cloud trailing her as usual, carrying a pet-carrier containing a tomcat I had neutered the prior week. Mrs. Wilson's face had that familiar smoldering glow of conflict about it. I feared I was about to endure yet another tirade.

From the treatment area I heard her snippy voice: "I want to speak with Dr. Slack. NOW!" The receptionist didn't have to come find me because Mrs. Wilson spoke so loudly she could be heard throughout the clinic.

I met her in the quiet room. "Hello, Mrs. Wilson, is there anything wrong?"

She didn't answer. Instead she opened the carrier and pulled out Mr. Tomcat and pointed at his scrotum with an accusatory expression plastered over her face as thick as the makeup she was wearing. "That's the problem, DOCTOR! And I don't think I should pay for such shabby work. I certainly will not pay for whatever you must do to save this poor orphan from your horrible mistake."

I looked where she was pointing. There, protruding from the tiny incision made when neutering, was a small piece of white tissue.

"My poor little baby has been licking "down there" and I am so worried and wondering why you did such a bad job! He's been in and out of his litter box, straining to relieve himself!"

I knew better then to suggest that maybe she should have brought him in a bit earlier. "I can certainly see why you are upset Mrs. Wilson. Let me keep him here until he's better."

"I don't expect to pay a penny more. This shouldn't have happened." With that said, she turned and left. I could hear her high heels clicking on the tile floor as she marched out the front door.

I took "Tom" back to the treatment area and examined the incision more closely. A sliver of fatty tissue was protruding from the incision. I gave a short-acting anesthetic, trimmed away the tissue and applied a soothing ointment. I secured an E-collar about his neck to keep him from licking "down there" and kept him in the treatment area where I could keep an eye on him. I decided it best to keep him overnight to be extra careful. I wanted nothing to rouse further ire in Tom's caretaker.

The next morning I removed the collar and continued to observe the cat to make sure he wasn't licking his scrotum or having difficulty urinating, remembering that Mrs. Wilson had mentioned he was "in and out of his litter box." He did just fine. No licking. No toilet problems. Nada.

Late in the afternoon the receptionist's voice came over the intercom. I couldn't help miss the sarcasm. "Dr. Bob, your favorite client Mrs. Wilson is on line one."

As I walked over to the phone I was thinking, I'll just nip this conversation in the bud. "Hello Mrs. Wilson," I said, not waiting for a reply before continuing, "Tom is doing just fine. He hasn't licked his scrotum all day and he hasn't had any difficulties urinating or defecating."

I felt quite smug as I waited for her reply. The line was silent for far too long. Finally I heard her take a deep breath before replying in her typical, loud condescending tone: "DR. SLACK, TOM IS MY HUSBAND. THE CAT'S NAME IS TOBY, NOT TOM!"

Click. The line went dead. I was mortified. I glanced down at "Tom's" medical record and sure enough, there at the bottom of the page plainly written under "pet's name" was Toby.

I was as red-faced as a vet could be after having assured a client that her husband was no longer licking his scrotum and was having normal bodily functions. There can be no recovery from such a gaffe.

My Master Communicator title – and attendant hubris – may have been shattered beyond repair, but there was a silver lining to the fall. I never saw Mrs. Wilson again. And my staff was well pleased at our loss of a client.

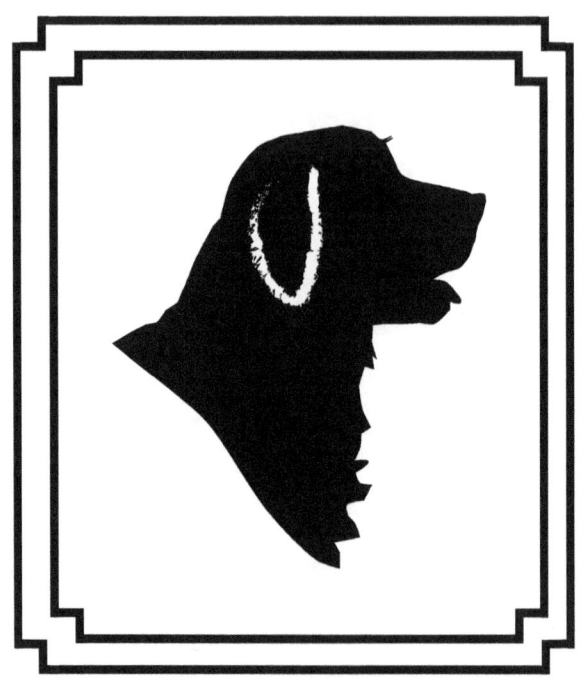

Monte & Bruce

Notwithstanding my disaster with Mrs. Wilson, I continued my part-time counseling career. And I became a better listener to my clients, animal and human.

Bruce was a loner. He was an "army brat," the son of a career soldier. His dad's frequent transfers made it difficult for Bruce to develop friendships. Just when he thought about befriending someone just to hang out with, another transfer would come along. He never had the chance to experience what a friendship felt like.

Bruce had just turned 15 when he entered his sophomore year in yet another school. He knew no one, but this was nothing new for him. It was just his life. He didn't feel he belonged. He thought of himself as an alien, and his physical features didn't help matters at all. His mom affectionately called him her "chubby little pal," which only applied more salt to his wounded self-image.

But he could deal with the bullying about his appearance most of the time: his family's constant military transfers had bred a certain toughness in him, thickened his skin. But there was one thing he could not protect himself from: the shower. This was his nightmare.

All P.E. kids were required to take group showers at his new school. Bruce suffered the terror over and over at "shower time" when the bullies exposed – and mercilessly mocked – the source of his fear. Bruce was slow to mature, and the bullies chose this to be the focus of their fun. They sensed his fear the way a predator senses wounded prey, and they gathered close about the shower room in anticipation of the P.E. bell that sounded the end of the period.

During P.E., Bruce would move as close as possible to the locker room, so when the bell rang he could be first to the shower, could let a few drops of water hit his naked body before he raced out to dress. He never made it. The bullies were onto his game, and they would intercept him coming out from the shower and humiliate him with their derogatory chants about his chubby body and lack of "manliness." He was mortified.

Bullying is one of the most destructive behaviors contrived by the human species for the sole purpose of inflicting pain upon another, whether that other is a human or a pet, in exchange for personal pleasure, or, as a bully might say, "just for the fun of it." That fun became pure pain for Bruce.

He was so deeply shamed that he vowed never to reveal the source of his pain. It drove his tears back inside him, and he vowed that he would never let anyone know how painful his life had become. He knew his tears would attract bullies as surely as flesh draws piranhas, and he used all his toughness to tuck away the damage they inflicted upon him.

His parents were the last ones he would tell. He feared his dad would storm the school in robust military fashion and then the whole school might find out why the bullies stalked him. He promised himself not to confide his fears to his mom, because he knew it would bring her to tears. She cried easily, and it always made him feel responsible for her sadness. She would never uncover his secret.

But there was a saving grace in his life: Monte, his golden

retriever. The after-school bus would drop Bruce off next to the dirt lane leading up to his home, and as soon as his feet hit the road he would see the graceful flash of a golden tail as Monte jumped off the porch and came bounding down the lane to meet him. Bruce would kneel down and run his hands through Monte's hair and stroke his fine head. Monte's delight in having his best friend home was met with such exuberance that you would have thought Bruce had been gone a lifetime.

Monte's whole demeanor was a roaring declaration of his devotion to Bruce, who knew deep down that he had in Monte somebody he could trust with his unspoken secret. He didn't need to "tell" Monte because it didn't matter. Monte accepted him unconditionally, and however his body looked, it was good enough for Monte.

Bruce felt like a whole person around Monte. Their time together gave him the strength to face each day's conflict in the communal shower. Monte made Bruce bully-proof, and helped him overcome one of the biggest challenges of his life. It was only years later that I learned of Monte from Bruce, who had become a client. By then I had returned to veterinary practice in Spokane.

Bruce had his third golden retriever, Rugar, put to sleep one evening at my veterinary hospital. The dog had lived to the grand old age of 16. I figured Rugar to be well into his 90s in human years. He died peacefully in Bruce's embrace. It was after hours so there was no hurry to rush off. Bruce had been coming to my clinic for 25 years, and we had become friends over time. I called the Pet Memorial Cemetery and they said they could pick up Rugar and would be by within the hour.

Bruce and I sat down by the coffee pot and it was then

that he told me about Monte. I have heard many stories through the years but this one was special. When I hear these "grace-filled" stories, I am reminded that there is something sacred to the bond between human and animal, between Bruce and Monte. The van arrived to take Rugar away, and as we watched the van pull away, Bruce turned to me and said, "You know Doc, I loved them all, but Monte was the best."

Monte got Bruce through those tough adolescent years. He matured, grew out of his chubby little body, and attended a prominent business college. He later married, had a couple of healthy kids and became an avid supporter of the local Humane Society. As I watched Bruce leave my clinic that night, I couldn't help wondering how things might have turned out without Monte to give Bruce the friendship he found missing from his early human world.

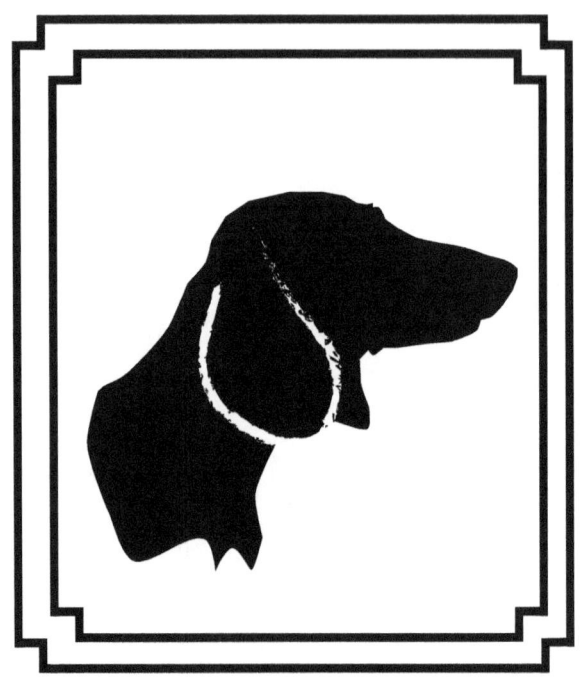

Sparks & Jeff

Jeff was an overachiever. He and his friends were approaching the final days of high school. They enjoyed teasing him for being selected as their class valedictorian. They liked his unpretentious nature, but they would never have guessed the chaos that ruled his home. He was so easy going that they never noticed he didn't talk about his home life, and Jeff always had such credible reasons for not inviting them to his house that the lack of invitations went unnoticed. He learned well how to mask his circumstances to keep his friends from uncovering the secret driving his need to overachieve. No one guessed that his father was a drunk.

Jeff's dad didn't drink every day. He had periods of sobriety when Jeff felt as if his family could be normal. Maybe, Jeff thought, it would be better if his dad drank all the time; that way Jeff wouldn't torture himself with false hope. That hope set him up for a greater fall whenever his dad suddenly and unpredictably went on another binge.

The change between Sober Dad and Drunk Dad was dramatic. When sober, his dad was interested in him. He became a part of the family: smiling, laughing, and spending time with Jeff woodworking in the garage. He genuinely liked this dad. But when a binge erupted, it unleashed another kind of dad. A nasty, raging, door-slammer who ranted himself into exhaustion. That dad would then retire to the TV room where he smoldered in dreadful silence, nursing a stiff drink. Jeff didn't have to guess if his dad was drinking in there. He could hear the ice clinking in the glass.

Jeff learned early on that bringing a friend home was to be avoided at all costs. The thought of the buddy seeing his dad drunk terrified him; he feared what might follow. He might be ridiculed, shunned or bullied as the son of a drunk. Just the thought would swamp him in a wave of shame.

Jeff imagined this must be what war is like, this constant state of readiness that never allowed him to let down his guard, even when he was away at school. He felt as if he were walking through a battlefield of hidden tripwires and land mines just waiting to be set off by his father's next alcoholic foray. The fragile ceasefire would suddenly evaporate into explosive chaos.

It was during those violent outbursts when Jeff's father would hurl hateful epithets at him, like shards of emotional shrapnel, wounding his youthful sensibilities. Jeff had no insulating vest to wrap around his heart to keep out the pain of his father's wounding words: "Grow up, you big baby. Quit your crying or I'll give you something to cry about. You're never going to amount to anything…"

After such episodes Jeff would steel himself with renewed determination to weather his dad's next binge, only to find himself once again helpless to dodge the pain of his father's harsh words. While these skirmishes never escalated to physical battles, when Jeff reflected years later on those dark times, he thought that perhaps verbal abuse was even worse than a physical attack.

There was simply no way to defend against the penetrating power of his father's words. He couldn't shut them out. While his father never laid a hand on him or never burst through his unlocked bedroom door, he hurled in his words. They echoed off the walls and ceilings, careened down the darkened hallway and smashed through his unopened door, filling his room with inescapable anger. It was if his father's anger was a ravenous beast that needed to be satisfied before it could slink back into the bottle it came from. During these tirades Jeff wished that he could will himself deaf just to shut out his father's wrath.

There were times of truce between binges, where Jeff experienced a reprieve from the abuse and he felt closer to his dad. But he knew better then to trust the calm between these storms. He was neither able to fully relax in the uncertainty of their relationship, nor able to lose hope that his dad might somehow escape the stranglehold booze had over him. In the midst of those turbulent times Jeff received a wonderful gift: Sparky.

Jeff remembered the exact day Sparky arrived. The pup was a present from his mom on his eighth birthday. He never understood how his mother had endured her husband's abuse but she must have recognized that a puppy might help her son deal with what she called her husband's "problem."

"Sparks," Jeff's name for his new friend, was a spunky little dachshund pup. Under the watchful eye of this long backed, short legged, feisty canine tutor, Jeff would find some semblance of normality in his life. Having him helped Jeff through his stormy childhood and teenage years, a time when tranquility was so fleeting that it seemed unreal, a figment of his imagination. Sparks was a welcome reprieve from the barbed tongue of his father's unearned criticism.

As Jeff neared the end of his high school days he began to think of his graduation as an announcement of freedom, a time to escape into another world, a more peaceful world.

He had a private celebration party with Sparks the day of his graduation, giving his loyal companion an edible diploma as an award for his faithfulness and as a promise that he would not abandon his best friend.

It was during Jeff's college years that I learned about his home life and how Sparks played such a vital role in helping him through those difficult years. He would bring Sparks into my clinic for his yearly check-up during his summer break. Jeff used to come with his mother all through his high school years, but now it was just he and Sparks. They were quite a couple. Sparks' tummy would sway from side to side as he waddled behind Jeff as they entered my exam room. Seeing them reminded me of a time when Jeff was still in high school. He and his mother brought Sparks in because he was in severe pain. Sparks cried out whenever they just touched him and howled if he thought they were about to touch him.

It turned out to be a serious problem. Sparks was eight years old at the time and had developed a problem with the discs between his vertebrae. One of these discs had "slipped" and put pressure on his spinal cord causing intense pain. Fortunately it did not progress to involve the muscles of the hind limbs, where, in the more serious cases, can even cause paralysis. The pain was bad enough.

It took several months of keeping Sparks confined and medicated for pain before he gradually recovered. But he would always be at risk for recurrence. Unfortunately this condition is not that uncommon to the dachshund breed.

During Sparks' convalescence, Jeff and his dad (during one of those welcomed sober stretches) built a ramp so Sparks could make it up onto Jeff's bed. I couldn't miss how important Sparks was to him. He became an excellent guardian for his pet's recovery, following my directions to the letter in caring for his companion.

Jeff's bond with Sparks was extraordinary. I mentioned this to Jeff and he laughed. "I remember how scared I was. That ramp was pretty cool. When Sparks got well enough to use it, he would crawl up under the covers at the foot of my bed. He liked being warm and would stay under there even during the summer. He would lie against my feet, keeping them warm in the winter but hot in the summer. I didn't care; I just enjoyed having a companion."

Following one of Sparks' annual visits during Jeff's college years, I invited him out for lunch to catch up on how life was treating him. That's when he told me his story, about how he and Sparks survived those early years living in an alcoholic home. He told me that Sparks, in a very real way, kept him from drowning in his father's verbal assaults. He did it by giving Jeff the perfect antidote: acceptance. And he gave it as only his species is capable of giving it: unconditionally, accepting him "just the way he was."

Jeff paused, his eyes tearing, before adding that his pet could never be a surrogate for his whole dad but he did provide the missing piece that his father could never provide. He confessed he longed for his father's approval and thought when he graduated class valedictorian, it might jog loose at least a speck of recognition. It didn't happen; his father remained mute, not acknowledging his son's academic accomplishments.

Jeff realized that part of his obsession to do well in school was an attempt to earn his father's approval. There is nothing more damaging to a young boy's self-worth than harsh, undeserved criticism delivered with anger. He now realized that it was his dog's total inability to criticize that was a major catalyst for their bond of friendship.

When he and Sparks took refuge in their bedroom to escape his father's rages, they became roommates seeking shelter from the storm. Because they had each other, it kept the walls of his room from closing in on him and becoming a prison. Sparks and Jeff transformed their room into a sanctuary, and their bond became a healing force.

"I think I grew closer to Sparks than most people do to their own pets because of my dad's drinking," Jeff said. "It drove us into the bedroom to escape the chaos that was always present whenever dad was home, even when he was sober the tension remained.

"Whenever I needed to retreat into the safety of my bedroom it was the presence of my pet that created a feeling that I had a home, a small home within our house. Within these walls Sparks and I took up our life together. It was here that I honed my academic skills that would reward me with the prestigious title of senior class valedictorian. A lofty title that did little to assuage my feeling I would never amount to much, those paternal words that would haunt me well after leaving home. Maybe it was Sparks that got me through it. In a crazy way, he became my mentor. I was calm with him next to me, I didn't worry so much, and that helped me concentrate."

"I don't totally understand what happened in that room. I'm a little embarrassed to tell you that Sparks and I learned how to talk to each other." He explained how they evolved their own unique way of communicating in a "wordless language," with nuanced tones, subtle movements and a magical quality of shared solitude.

Jeff began to ascribe meaning to Sparks' sounds, vocalizations and subtle movements, expanding their personal shared vocabulary. He noticed how Sparks also picked up on his own voice tones and movements, keeping the conversation flowing both ways. Jeff especially singled out the inexplicable fluency that spilled unspoken meaning from the eyes of his canine companion. Jeff was obviously quite proud of what he considered their rather highly evolved form of "inter-species" conversation, yet, at the same time reserved in his boasting for fear I might think him a bit "odd."

I laughed to myself, thinking how often I have heard so many clients through the years talk about their own pets "special" way of understanding them, even to the point they had to resort to spelling certain words to keep their pet from deciphering what they were actually saying. One client in particular had to be careful not to say "vet" on the day of their scheduled visit to my clinic to avoid spending the morning trying to extract her toy poodle from beneath the bed.

I mentioned to Jeff that I knew dogs could detect fear from my own experience as a veterinarian, and, as a pet owner, I knew my own pets could detect other emotions as well. Jeff nodded, adding that Sparks could detect some of his emotions as well, naming anxiety and anger among them.

"When I was angry, Sparks would retreat to his favorite rug in the corner of the room. With his head between his outstretched paws, he would follow me about the room, moving only his eyes, following my every movement, his body completely still while he waited out my stubborn surliness.

Sparks had superhuman patience waiting out Jeff's anxiety

and anger.

"The moment when he sensed that my mood had finally turned, he would suddenly jump up and scamper around and around the room as if in celebration of anger's retreat. Then the room would fill with my laughter. When I was happy, Sparks would drum out a lively tune with his tail. I called it Sparks' "happy tail."

"When I talked, Sparks listened. In fact, he listened very attentively, as if sensitive to the nuanced feel of my many moods, and he responded with behaviors that resonated with those moods. Sparks would sometimes sit directly in front of me…staring, giving me the distinct feeling I was being heard, and even understood."

Sparks came to know Jeff's moods so well that he developed empathetic responses: a wild tail wag for excitement, a soft tail wag for contentment, a whimper for worry, and a nose-bump for frustration that seemed to say, "I'm bored. Can't we do something else?"

Jeff felt confident that he could distinguish the meaning of a great array of different "signals" Sparks gave him. He was especially taken by Sparks' subtle, almost inaudible whimper, which seemed to say: "Ah yes, go on, say more. Makes sense to me!"

As I listened to Jeff's explanations of how they communicated with each other, I realized it was not important how credible I thought his story was because it was quite evident that whatever they did seemed to work well for them.

Sparks had an uncanny ability to coax Jeff out of his funky moods as if he recognized the futility of it all. In his darker moments, Sparks would race to the closet and retrieve the red ball that Jeff called their "attitude adjustment" ball.

"But Sparks just called it 'woof,'" said Jeff. "He would pad over to me and gently deposit the ball in my outstretched hand to begin a game of fetch that went on until exhaustion – either human or canine – rang the closing bell."

Sparks also schooled Jeff in the art of listening. Years later, his girlfriend told him that he was such a wonderful listener, making her feel that she was very important, that he really cared about what she was saying. She said that at these times she felt especially close to him. "I just smiled and answered, 'my dog taught me how to listen'. She just stared at me in stunned disbelief, thinking I must be teasing her, testing her gullibility."

What would life have been like without Sparks? Jeff's room would have been a prison, he would have fallen into a depression, and retreated inside himself to shut out a dangerous world.

Jeff took Sparks with him to college. A few of his professors recognized the importance of this well-behaved, aging dachshund to their bright student, and they allowed Sparks to accompany Jeff to some of their classes.

Sparks had a good life. Jeff brought him in to see me each summer during the young man's college years for the little dog's checkups and vaccinations. Sparks is 14 years old at the time of this writing, and still trucking along – although his tummy now scrapes along the ground, a consequence of the distance between his front and hind legs.

Recently, I gave Sparks his annual checkup and was relieved to note that his back was holding up quite well. It was during this checkup that I learned how college life was treating Jeff. He was making a good life for himself, and he would not be following in the footsteps of his father. It's not easy to break away from such a legacy: the tentacles of alcoholism go deep, strangling the family with shame and infecting it with an insidious tendency to replicate. Jeff made his escape by breaking the family's sad legacy with the help of a fiery little friend named Sparks.

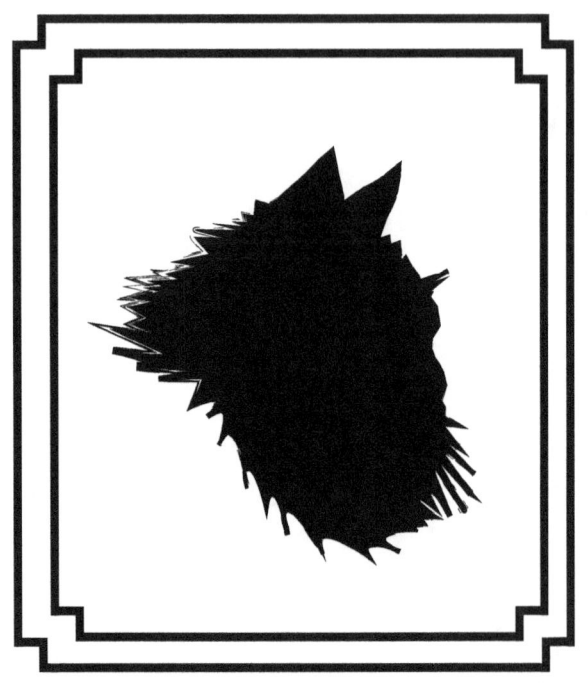

Pearl & Marge

Pearl and Marge taught me that the bond can be so powerful that not even death can stop a guardian's commitment to his or her animal's welfare.

Marge wore a scarf, blue with white polka dots, drawn tightly around her head. Her face is pale, her eyes tired. An emptiness had replaced the lively sparkle so familiar from previous visits. Her spunky personality had drained away, as though pressed out by some great weight. The scarf couldn't hide her grief. It merely covered the rude intrusion of her chemotherapy and its merciless assault upon her femininity.

I want to respect her privacy, and I try to restrain myself from glancing at her scarf. I have failed, because her eyes suddenly fall. We say nothing; her eyes ask me not to ask. I break the pregnant silence. "You're a bit early for Pearl's annual visit, Marge."

"I know. I just want to be sure she's okay, that nothing's wrong with her." I wonder if this is about the scarf.

On the exam table sits Pearl, a sullen fluffy white Persian cross. She is my perennial crank and nemesis. We accepted years ago our mutual dislike. Each year she takes her position in the center of the exam table and glares at me, as if she's waiting to see who blinks first. Pearl knows she is in control, and I know her glare is no bluff. I have never reconsidered taking her temperature after our initial battle, when she was yet a wee kitten.

I (obviously) lost that battle, which set the tone for

our subsequent visits in which I am forced to accept her dominance. I'm bothered by the fact that Pearl knows I am the one who always backs down. There is more than a subtle hint of arrogance in the way she dismisses me with her low, prolonged growl, punctuated with a sudden hiss at the end as if she even needed an exclamation mark to prove her superiority. Pearl uses her nasty disposition to keep her annual exams brief and, I'm embarrassed to admit, not at all thorough.

Even her size is intimidating. She tips the scale at a glorious 18 pounds. At least nine of them are due to her being overweight; the other nine are pure attitude. If I am not misinterpreting her behavior, she's damned proud of it, too.

Pearl has been stuck at this weight forever. One year, to encourage Marge to put Pearl on a diet, I used my impressive medical approach. I like to think it's powerfully persuasive. It failed miserably. Last year I tried benign manipulation, but both Marge and Pearl saw through that one, too.

Marge tolerates my annual diet lectures; she nods politely as she listens to my "doctor talk" about the many hazards of Pearl's condition. I fool myself into thinking she has been persuaded to cut back on the groceries, but in my heart I know Pearl runs the show at home, as well. Anyway, Marge puts up with me. She knows my intentions are good. But I see that today is not a time to discuss Pearl's portliness.

The truth is that there is not much I can do with Pearl. Taking her temperature is only the first in a list of the things I cannot do. A dental exam consists of waiting for her to do one of her snarly hisses so I can glimpse her teeth from a safe distance. Listening to her heart only results in a "too quick to be seen" swat from her front paw with its razor-sharp claws. And forget probing that fluffy tummy; that would only insult her delicate sensibilities and ramp up her indignation. To be honest, Pearl is one cat I am actually terrified of, and she knows it. I would feel safer examining a rabid Rottweiler.

My exam deteriorates into a question-and-answer period. I ask the questions; Marge answers and Pearl glares.

"How's her appetite, Marge?" I can't believe I lead with that particular question. It's one of those hated moments when I can actually see the words leaving my mouth, with no way in hell to stop them from filling the room with my insensitivity.

"Fine," she says. I wisely avoid pursuing a follow-up question, like "What does 'fine' mean in this case?" Besides, it seems to me that she said "fine" with a hint of sarcasm in her tone. But maybe I am being a bit defensive.

"Does she have normal bowel movements?"

"Yes."

"Is she lethargic?" I ask this knowing from past answers that if Pearl were to sleep any more, additional hours would have to be allotted to each day.

I hesitate to ask Marge about the cat's water consumption. I live in fear that at one of our visits her answer might be "It's excessive." This is one of the signs of diabetes (a companion to obesity) which would trigger the need for both a more thorough exam and a blood draw!

I can't imagine a more difficult task than teaching Marge how to give insulin injections if her cat were to become diabetic. To say that Pearl would be a formidable foe would be a wild understatement, painful for everyone involved.

"Is she drinking more water than normal?"

"No, same as always." Ah, a pardon.

After a few more inquiries I confirm that Pearl's history has not changed in any significant way. I begin to suspect that Marge is not here because of anything specific about Pearl's health. She just seems to need reassurance that Pearl is okay. I'm not too concerned about my lack of thoroughness, because I sense that Marge is here for a different reason, but I'm unsure how to approach changing the course we're on.

"Marge, I think Pearl is just fine. Six years old is still on the young side of life. I could sedate her to give her a proper physical. We could run some lab tests, but since you haven't noticed any change in her health from her behavior at home, I don't think that's necessary."

She nods answering, "You're right, she's hasn't changed her usual habits at home." With some apprehension, I ask, "Are you worried about anything in particular?"

Marge is silent. Our eyes meet, and I see tears beginning in hers. She looks frightened as she blurts out, "Do you think Pearl has cancer?"

There it is, out in the open. I have seen this before, when a client is diagnosed with a particular problem, he or she will sometimes begin to worry about a pet's health. I know Marge trusts me, and I decide to use this trust to quell her fear. Perhaps that's all I can do today, give her reassurance.

"She looks good, Marge. You have always taken such good care of her. Your annual checkups were done on time, she's up on her vaccinations, you haven't reported anything today that makes me suspect she has cancer, or any other disease, for that matter." Nodding her head, she smiles for the first time.

Marge reaches over and strokes Pearl under her chin, dabs

her own eyes with a handkerchief she has retrieved from her purse, and replies, "Thank you. I just wanted to make sure." She looks less worried.

She opens the door to the carrier, and Pearl squeezes herself through the opening. Marge laughs, "I fight with her to get her in this darn contraption coming, but she has no problem getting herself in when it's time to go!"

I sense that our time for now is over. I have gotten to know Marge quite well over the years. She has always been chatty, but I understand her reticence and I will not pry. I end our meeting with, "Marge, I want you to call me if you notice anything about Pearls behavior that worries you." She nods and assures me she will let me know if she notices anything that concerns her.

Several weeks pass after my meeting with Marge and Pearl, I notice that a new client has made an appointment to see me. The receptionist lets me know that she just wants to meet me. I think nothing of it. More and more these days, new clients want to visit our hospital and meet us before actually deciding to bring in their pets.

I enter the exam room, and the new client rises from her seat holding out her hand. "Hi, Dr. Slack. My name is Mary. We have mutual friends, Marge and her cat, Pearl. She gave Pearl to me to care for, and she wanted you to continue being Pearl's doctor."

I am caught off guard by her statement. My mind hasn't caught up with what I am feeling. "Glad to meet you, Mary. How is Marge doing?"

She looks startled. "I am really sorry, Doctor, I thought you knew. Marge passed on just last week."

I think back to our last time together. I grasp why she came in that day; she was setting her house in order. She needed reassurance that Pearl was okay. It might have been the last link in her chain of concerns before handing her beloved cat over to this lady standing before me.

"I didn't know she was that ill. I knew she was sick, but I saw her only a few weeks ago. She must really trust you, Mary, to give over to you her best friend." Mary's eyes tear up and she nods, "Marge and I have been friends for many years." Usually I lose my favorite clients when their pets pass on and they decide not to have any more. This is different. I think Marge's suffering must have been lessened knowing Pearl was healthy and Mary would be there to give her a new home. She needed to know that Pearl would not be left homeless or ill. Finding a "foster mom" must have been her last remaining task, freeing her from worry, giving her permission to pass in peace.

Several months after I met Mary, my thoughts returned to Marge and our long history together, one born of her love for a cranky cat who apparently won't be going away anytime soon. The loss of Marge had softened my thoughts regarding Pearl. Marge entrusted her feline companion to me, and I felt a guilt-driven obligation to care for Pearl, a curious application of the Hippocratic oath in which "do no harm" must work both ways.

I start to see Pearl through Marge's eyes. I know that Pearl has a soft side to her schizoid nature, which could instantly transform from tyrannical bully into submissive sweetness by the mere stroke of Marge's finger to the underside of Pearl's chin. That simple touch had the power to quell the rage that surfaced in Pearl at the mere sight of me entering the exam room.

Pearl's body had relaxed to the sound of Marge's voice purring, "That's my girl. Be good for Dr. Bob." But those feline eyes never left me; they fixed me with an unwavering, unsettling stare. It was Pearl's wordless way of letting me know that I was not Marge, and I would be made to pay for that oversight.

There were brief moments of civility that gave me insight into Marge's incredible attachment to Pearl. I did my best to respect the bond between them by attending to Pearl's health in spite of our differences.

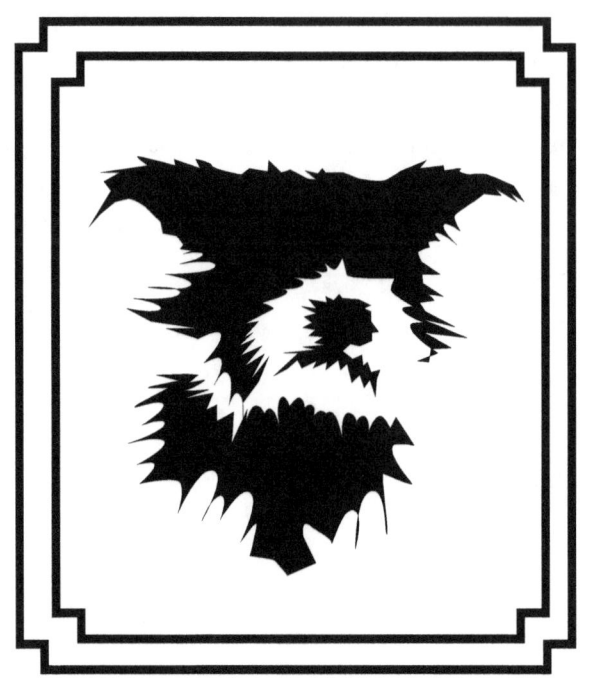

Juno & James

The best of intentions can sometimes get in the way of providing the care our pets need. Most pets love to eat, and most guardians love the way feeding reinforces the bond between them. Feeding the bond can become a problem when love (and guilt) clouds our judgment. The story of Juno and James is a perfect cautionary tale of too much of a good thing. Fortunately, this tale has a happy ending.

James was new to our clinic. He was an out-of-towner. He said that a friend had recommended that he come see me about his dog, Juno, a large mixed-breed male lying next to him. Before James said a word about what brought him in to see me, I knew that the problem would in some way relate to Juno's condition: extreme obesity. Before I even introduced myself, my new client began explaining his problem.

"Doc, I don't know what to do about my dog. He can't get up anymore without my help. He wants to. He tries, but can't get up. I take a towel and put it around his belly and lift him up; that's the only way he can make it. This morning he messed himself before I could get him outside."

At that point, James covered his face with his hands and sobbed. I waited. After composing himself, he continued. "I've been going to this vet near my place, but all he says is I gotta get Juno's weight down. I've tried but he just won't lose any weight. I've really tried."

I didn't know what he meant by "I've tried," but I did

know that James was as sincere as he was distraught. He talked about how he and Juno lived alone on a small farm outside Clayton, a small town near us in eastern Washington State. He explained that he had always had a dog in his life. But Juno was different. Juno was "one in a million."

The more James talked, the more I liked him. There was a simple, honest openness about him. He talked for several more minutes, telling me the various things he had tried to get Juno to lose weight, things either he'd thought of or the other vet had suggested.

I stooped down next to Juno. He lifted his muzzle off the floor and stared back at me. Some dogs don't like to look directly at you, but Juno did. He had that gentle stare, the kind of look that just feels soft, the kind that makes you feel comfortable. I held out the back of my hand and he sniffed it, paused, and then licked my fingers. His tail gave a single lazy thump and then fell quiet. Juno had won me over. I thought of James' words, "He's one in a million."

I looked up at James and said, "Let's see if we can help." I said "we" because I knew that regardless of what I came up with for a diagnosis, it would need to include diet as part of the plan. And that part would rest with James.

I gave Juno a thorough physical, and I could turn up no obvious problems other than excess weight, muscle wasting and tenderness in the hips. I suspected his muscle wasting was due to limited exercise, again related to the obesity. I suspected arthritis as the source of the hip pain, which would certainly contribute to the old fellow's difficulty in getting up by himself and his not wanting to walk. Also, at nine, Juno was no longer a young dog. Nine is in the senior-citizen range for a dog of his size, and this also contributed to the problem.

I asked James if I could keep Juno for the rest of the day. I could tell that my request made him a bit nervous, but after I explained what I wanted to do he agreed – as long as he could come back later that day to take him home. I also got permission to call his other vet. When James gave me the vet's name, I realized that I knew him.

Later that day I had my colleague on the line. "Say, Tom, I had James in with Juno this morning, and…" Tom broke in with a chuckle, "So, James came to see you. Nice guy. Doesn't like the word 'diet,' though!" He then filled me in on the blood work he had recently run on Juno. "Perfect," he replied. "Not a single chemistry out of line."

I was especially concerned about a low thyroid test, but Juno's thyroid function was perfectly normal. And his blood sugar and liver enzymes were all in the middle of normal. Tom had also taken x-rays of the dog's back and hips, which revealed arthritis in his spine and in both hips.

After talking with Tom a bit longer, I hung up. I decided to repeat the thyroid test just to confirm his conclusion. There's nothing worse than trying to get an untreated low-thyroid pet to lose weight by dieting. It's like pushing a truck up a hill with a chain.

James came in later that afternoon, and I reviewed the conversation I'd had with Tom, explaining why I was repeating the thyroid test. I thought it best to wait for the results. I could see the apprehension in James' eyes, "You think you can help Juno?" "Maybe WE can," I replied. James looked at me and smiled, the first sign of hope I'd seen from him. "Oh, yeah, Doc, I forgot. You have this thing about 'we.'"

Several days later the test results confirmed Tom's conclusion: normal thyroid function. I had our receptionist give James a call to come in to see me.

"James," I began, "I think we can help Juno. I'm not sure, but I do think there is a good chance we can get him back on his feet again. But I'm not sure about you. I'm not sure you can follow my advice."

James looked hurt. "Doc, I would do anything if I felt it would help Juno."

"I want you to hear me out, then," I said. "I am going to ask you to do something I don't think you will want to do." He looked at me, puzzled. I went on. "I told you I think we can get Juno back on his feet, but to do that I will be asking you to do something that will be very hard for you."

"What's that?"

"To help Juno, I will want you to cut back on the amount of food you are feeding him. But if you do that, Juno is going to make you feel very guilty, maybe even cruel. I'm wondering if you can deal with that."

James looked stunned. "Doc, I have cut back on his food already. Honest. It doesn't work. Something else is wrong with him, I'm sure."

"Look, James, I know you've tried. Dr. Larsen told me that you've tried. But I wonder if you think you're being mean when you cut back on his groceries."

James fell silent. He stared at the floor for a while. "I never thought of it that way," he said. "Juno loves to eat, and when I started feeding him less, he would bang his empty food dish with his paw and look up at me with that look."

I knew just what James meant by "that look."

"I would give him just a little more, but I guess maybe my 'little' was a bit too much," said James.

I brought out a dish and a bag of dog food and asked James to show me how much food he fed on average and how frequently he fed Juno. My assumption was correct: James was feeding Juno almost twice the amount of food he needed to maintain him in his obese state.

Weight loss was out of the question for Juno if James kept up that routine. I showed James the amount of food I thought would be necessary to begin a weight-loss program. He looked at me with disbelief written all over his face. I laughed, "James, you are not a bad person. You're just a victim of your own soft heart. I can't beat you up for caring for Juno, but you are going to have to learn a different way of caring for him – a way other than food. To do this, you have to understand that cutting back on the food is what's best for Juno, even though it doesn't feel right. Are you following me?

"In putting him on a diet, you will also be helping him with his arthritis. I think I'll give you some pain medication for that, as well. When his weight comes down, you may not even need to continue the medication. We just have to wait to see about that."

He slowly nodded and looked up, and with a voice of resignation, he said, "This is going to be very hard on me, Doc." I believed him because I also heard the sound of surrender in his reply, a sign that we just might be taking a tentative step in the right direction.

I believe that in many cases of obesity, the approach to helping a guardian accept the idea of dieting is to let him or her know that you understand how difficult this is emotionally. Reducing a pet's food is usually accompanied with strong feelings of guilt. Many folks use food to nurture the bond they have with their pet; therefore, to ask them to pull back on the food is the same as asking them not to love their pet so much.

This approach may also be silently telling them they are bad people for letting their pets get into this situation in the first place. They may feel doubly guilty. First for watching their pets go hungry (which looks to them like starving), and second for not being able to stop overfeeding their pets.

Guilt, if it goes unrecognized, can sometimes sabotage a diet program. I will ask a client directly if she sometimes feels guilty when it comes to her pet's weight problem. I am not surprised when the client's eyes well up with tears, and she says, "I do feel guilty, but those sad eyes just get to me and I give in. I know I shouldn't, but I just can't help myself. I know it is selfish of me, but I get pleasure out of feeding my pet."

When I hear this confession, it gives me an opportunity to validate the client's feelings and to ask a critical question: "Do you think you can keep your pet on a diet in spite of feeling the way you do – knowing that by helping your pet lose weight you will be protecting his or her health?" I am encouraged when they respond with, "Thank you, Doctor. You're the first vet to understand how hard it is for me to feed my pet less." I reply, "I would not ask you to do this if I didn't believe in the long run it is the best thing we can do for his or her health."

That last sentence will fall on deaf ears if it's not preceded by an acknowledgment of how difficult it can be to put one's beloved pet on a diet. A little sincere empathy can go a very long way when it comes to dieting.

A client's response to guilt is unpredictable. For some, guilt is too painful, so they become angry. Sometimes this anger comes out openly, as in, "How come all you vets think Fifi's fat? I think she's just fine the way she is. I just want you to fix her back problem."

More frequently I get the passive side of anger, "Okay, Dr. Bob. I'll cut back on her food." But I know that the client is really thinking, "The next time I come in, I'm going to ask for Dr. Wellon. He doesn't bring up Fifi's weight, because her weight really isn't that bad. Dr. Slack just has this 'thing' about weight!"

It would be wrong of me to put the entire blame on the guardian. Pets have very creative ways of instilling guilt in their guardians. Some carry their food dish around the house, dropping it at their guardian's feet or banging it around the hardwood floor. This direct approach is frequently successful.

Other pets take a more subtle approach, sitting in front of their guardian and staring intently, occasionally smacking their lips, allowing a pathetic string of drool to dangle sympathetically before the weaker of the two species, "guilting" him into submission.

Cats like to use the vocal approach, sitting in front of the fridge yowling pitifully. In this situation, feeding is done not in sympathy but as the only way to shut the #@&*! cat up. Some cats like to do the obsessive leg-rubbing thing. They turn and twist from one guardian ankle to the other until, magically, food appears.

Sulking also can be effective. Somehow a dog or cat might learn that if she acts depressed, food will suddenly appear. Some pets appear to know intuitively that their guardian is hopelessly codependent. I would not be surprised if "Over-Feeders Anonymous" groups were to arise in the future to help with this "feeding the bond" syndrome. The hidden message from our very smart pets is this: "If you don't feed me as often as I would like to be fed, I will not like you: you are a very bad guardian."

The tricks pets learn in order to cadge food from their gullible owners are numerous. So it isn't totally the fault of the guardian that his pet's belly begins its sad pilgrimage to the floor. One time I put Abby, my first yellow Lab, on a strict diet. A month later I noticed she had gained weight. I live out in the country, and it wasn't until a neighbor a mile away called to tell me that Abby had become a frequent visitor that I figured out the problem. The neighbors fed their dog by leaving a bag of food open in the garage so that their pet could partake whenever he felt the urge.

This works for some pets, but it didn't work AT ALL with a Labrador named Abby. She stopped eating only when her stomach was stretched to the point of bursting. I had to kennel Abby, and I couldn't even take her for a walk off lead because she would vanish somewhere along the way, only to return after she had obviously located a cache of food somewhere in the hinterlands. Never underestimate a retriever's nose: it is much more reliable in locating food than a car's GPS is at finding a street address. Sadly, confinement was the only solution to keeping Abby on a diet. And yes, I felt guilty.

My own experience and that of my other clients make me confident that James' attachment to Juno would be the root of the problem. He confessed that he felt incredibly guilty and sad when he made Juno diet, and this was the principal reason why he had been unable to stick to the regimen recommended by the other vet. He realized that he'd minimized the role of weight in his pet's difficulty in getting up and walking. He blamed Juno's pain and immobility on arthritis, and he was angry with his other vet for not focusing more on the arthritis instead of the dog's weight.

I told James that I felt weight played the greater role in Juno's difficulties, but I would never neglect his dog's pain. I put Juno on a strict diet and made James use a measuring cup to keep him from "cheating." He agreed to my Gestapo tactics.

James came three weeks later for a recheck and I noticed immediately that Juno had lost weight. I praised James for holding his ground. I came up with an approximate target weight of 70 pounds. Juno began dieting at the grand weight of 120 pounds and graced the scales with a nice drop of 5 pounds to 115!

Over the next 10 months, Juno lost an incredible 45 pounds. It wasn't easy on either pet or guardian. I had James bring Juno in weekly for several weeks and then monthly over the final six-month period for weigh-ins and to see how Juno's ambulation was coming along. When Juno reached his target weight he looked terrific!

More important were the other changes that came with the weight loss. "Doc, you can't believe how he's doing," said James. "He's like a new dog, like he was when he was younger. He has his energy back, and, you know, I don't think his arthritis is even bothering him."

I could see that Juno's muscle mass had increased as he'd become more active. One of the obvious complications of obesity is the fact that it is frequently accompanied by lethargy, and in Juno's case, compounded by arthritis. Now that his weight was in the normal range and his muscle tone had improved dramatically, his arthritis seemed to have magically disappeared, and we were able to wean him off pain meds. I knew that his arthritis pain would probably return as he aged, but he didn't need medications again until a couple of years later.

Working with clients on weight loss for their pets can be very trying at times, and the success I had with Juno has helped me to be persistent and patient in working with this particular problem that veterinarians face all too frequently.

Remembering the excitement on James' face when he exclaimed, "He's like a new dog!" and seeing Juno prance up to the scale for that final weigh-in has served me well in my efforts to remain steadfast in encouraging others to nurture their pets in ways other than feeding. Most clients already know if their pet's weight is a serious problem; they just need encouragement and understanding about how difficult it is to learn alternative ways to nurture the bond.

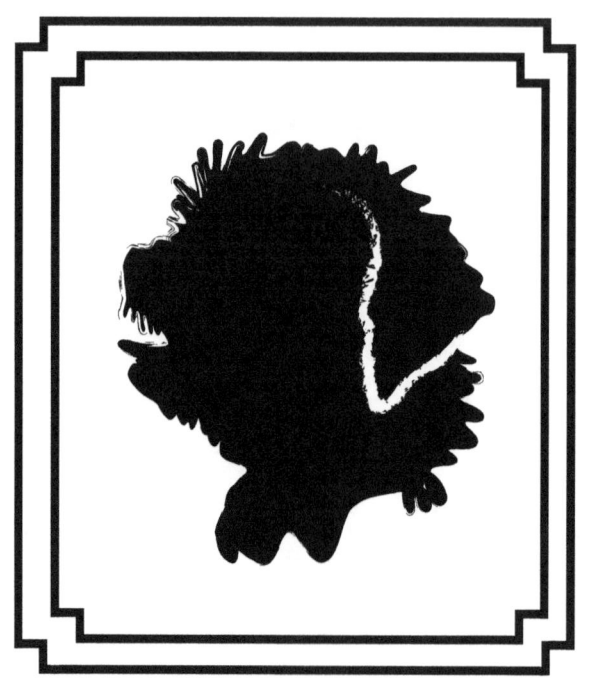

Sadie & Shane

My experience as a vet – and the shared experience with clients and their pets – has taught me an enormous amount about the bond. There is also a parallel learning about the bond between humans and animals that takes place in families. The bond grows as we tell stories about our pets and share them as a family – how pets become family members, the joy they bring, and the lessons they teach about being alive, getting old and dying.

Pets, like humans, have their favorites in the family. Although I brought Sadie the Shih Tzu home and our whole family bonded with her, she chose our son Shane as her human best friend. Pet owners know what outsize roles our pets play in family dynamics. Given Sadie's compact size, the impact of her reign seemed that much greater. A little background before exploring that bond with Shane will help explain her dominance.

Some folks believe the Shih Tzu came to humanity unnaturally. They think the breed was fashioned by a committee, a cadre of artists in some trendy studio where humor over function was the guiding principle. They back up this claim by pointing out the many odd characteristics of this breed, and they question to which species the Shih Tzu really belongs. They suggest that perhaps it is a species onto itself – a confused species that couldn't decide if it wanted to be cat or dog.

On the cat side of the species dispute, it has a vague resemblance to the Persian, while on the dog side it risks being ridiculed as the "tiny odd one" because of its natural physical peculiarities: short legs, a serious underbite, a pushed-in snout, a tongue meant for a dog four times its size, dangerously protruding eyes, and a proud tail that feathers over the back leaving the dog's bum arrogantly exposed. And, like its big shorthaired brother, the bulldog, a Shih Tzu cannot breathe quietly.

As a veterinarian, I am well aware of these oddities and the medical issues that arise from them. Unfortunately, "odd" in veterinary language becomes "anomaly," and anomalies can sometimes cause health problems. So what did this vet do after familiarizing himself with this breed's anomalies? I went out and adopted one. Before judging me too harshly, let me defend myself.

Her name is Sadie. She came into our home with all the oddities of her breed, but she also came with another trait typical of her breed: an abundance of contagious joy. She instantly "infected" my family with her winsome personality, and our bond with her was forged in a heartbeat. It was not wisdom, but rather foolishness that led me to adopt such an unusual little creature. But the spell she cast over our entire human family was inescapable.

We people greeted her with excitement, but Bailee, my black-and-white Springer Spaniel, and Shilo, my yellow Lab, emphatically did not. I say my, because even though they are family dogs, they are also mine. Perhaps I should say I am theirs, just as Shane was Sadie's. But I am getting ahead of myself.

I carefully placed the twelve-week-old puppy between the big dogs, alert to how they would handle the presence of their strangely-shaped new roommate, then slowly backed away to take in the whole picture of my animal trio. I think profound disbelief – mixed with disgust – best describes the look on their faces.

In the early weeks of Sadie's life I would carry her to work in my coat pocket. She loved the clinic, not minding being placed in a kennel for part of each day. She delighted in being spoiled by all the attention from staff and clients, but spurned any attempts by her own kind to socialize with her.

I believe she thought herself completely human. In contrast, my hunting dogs straddled two worlds. They played with each other, stayed close to each other outdoors, slept together and became anxious if separated. When I was present, however, they ignored each other and turned all their attention to me. Sadie, though, was completely comfortable with her exclusively human identity. She shunned her giant siblings all the days of her life.

Our girl had her day in the sun when I took her with me to do a weekly TV program. The program featured segments on current animal care problems and special interest stories involving pets. The first morning I brought Sadie to the TV station she was only three months old. She sat on my lap, chewing on my finger. The woman interviewing me was so enamored with Sadie that she focused totally on her, asking about her breed and age and gushing over her cuteness. Sadie became the star and I was demoted to second banana. When I stopped bringing her to the studio, the station canceled the program. Go figure.

Despite her size, Sadie knew that she was a force to be reckoned with, and displayed almost cat-like control over us with advanced expertise in manipulating humans. We fed her on her command and we opened and closed doors on her command. She barked to summon us to play with her. In other words, she owned us, or perhaps more accurately, ruled over us humans as well as her much larger canine siblings.

Because of her highly developed manipulative skills, I mostly remember Sadie as clever, except when she caught sight of her canine siblings. I don't know what it is about small breeds, but they frequently have a big-dog complex that causes them to act like morons and attack dogs ten times their size.

There was neither a smidgen of insight nor a remnant of instinct in her little body to warn her that size really does matter. The inability to evaluate risk in this particular area is common – and unfortunate – in the smaller breeds. I should know, after all the little dogs who have found their way onto my surgery table to have their "wounds of ignorance" closed. Sadly, serious wounds have little effect in stopping future episodes of aggression. Sadie escaped injury only because of my vigilance, but she had some very close calls. More than once, I snatched her from the jaws of a giant.

One episode stands out: the time I stepped out our front door to see a mangy coyote with a very hungry look standing directly in front of Sadie and only a leap away. True to her "big-dog" affliction, Sadie was oblivious to the danger, barking and growling ferociously. It would have been comical had it not been nearly fatal.

The coyote stood like a tightly wound spring, glancing at me before returning to stare at its prey. Its gaunt appearance and unnatural lack of fear suggested he was a very hungry animal indeed. He reacted to Sadie's antics as though they were a polite invitation to an uncooked dinner. I was alarmed by his total disregard of my presence – and Sadie's reveling in playing her imagined role as puffed-up family protector.

I occasionally worried about coyotes that sometimes visited our forested acreage, but many months had passed with nary a sign of these wily predators, and I had dropped my guard. I thought letting Sadie out to do her business was quite safe, but at this moment I was proven completely wrong. We'd had an unusually severe winter that year that must have driven these wild members of the canine family to range closer to their domestic food source: tiny dogs and other small animals. Coyotes feel no guilt in consuming close relatives, and Sadie was, at this very moment, as close as a coyote's relative can be and still be alive.

I leaped off the porch, giving out a yell as I ran toward Sadie. I was the unwanted dinner guest, an uninvited intruder into what I am sure the interloper thought was a done deal. Again, the coyote turned its lazy gaze toward me and then slowly turned and loped toward the woods, stopping every few steps along the way to turn and stare back at its lost dinner before moving on. It was then that I saw its hunting partner appear from behind a stand of trees. They trotted toward one other and slowly disappeared, like ghosts, into the woods.

Unfortunately, Shilo and Bailee reinforced Sadie's delusional behavior. They became cowards in her presence, backing down from her bluster, allowing their tiny sister to bully them, reinforcing the misperception that all big dogs would fear her. If she didn't want them smelling her butt, she would spin around at lightning speed, growling as fiercely as a puffball can growl, then lunge at them, her teeth making staccato sounds as they gnashed sharply together. She had

Shilo and Bailee totally buffaloed. Sadie became the undisputed alpha female of the entire household.

Sadie's "big dog complex" reminds me of another equally moronic syndrome, one that she thankfully did not inherit. I call it the "Porcupine Revenge Syndrome." This pathetic condition is characterized by the inability of dogs to refrain from re-attacking porcupines even after they've encountered the incredible pain guaranteed by such an attack. In fact, the more quills per-square-inch embedded in a dog's nose, tongue, throat, and paws, the greater the seeming likelihood that the dog will seek out another quill donor. These dogs obviously lack the common sense gene and get classed with big dog complex sufferers.

There is little hope of eliminating the genes responsible for these "defective" behaviors because we humans cannot resist being lured into a bond with dogs as surely as sailors could not resist being drawn onto the rocks by the mythical sirens. And so we humans travel back and forth, from home to vet hospital, to patch up our animals' wounds so that they may pass their defective genes on to their posterity.

There may be another as yet unidentified gene at play in a dog's – or for that matter – a cat's ability to select from a group which human will be their favored one. It is usually the one most likely to meet their needs. Sadie was very astute in selecting our son Shane to be her best friend, her chosen one. She picked him over me, my wife Lois, and the other children in our family. The bond between Shane and Sadie would run long and deep.

She quickly had him wrapped around her little paw. He became her companion and protector. Shane fed her, played with her and fretted over her, noticing any small change in her behavior and bringing problems to my attention. He was the perfect guardian for her.

Sadie blessed Shane in turn by taking her undesired traits elsewhere. One in particular comes to mind – the gift of the poop fairy – and you don't have to lose a tooth to receive the Tootsie Roll. This fairy never deposited her gifts in Shane's room. That was sacred ground. My bedroom, on the other hand, became her favorite depository. I first learned of this in the dead of night while stumbling in the dark to my own depository. Tootsie Rolls stick nicely between human toes, and you don't even need to turn the lights on to know the poop fairy has blessed you with her gift.

Animal behaviorists call this unfortunate behavior "incomplete house training," and they believe that its cause is incompetent people in charge of a dog's training. That would be me. I think that in my case you would have to add laziness to the mix. I offer a word of professional caution: do not be lazy. Once the behavior becomes entrenched, it is doubly hard to extinguish.

Small dogs tend to be more likely "incompleters." I suggest you be diligent in following proven routes to finishing and reinforcing your dog's house training. Always follow the advice of a veterinarian, because you know vets are infallible experts, especially when it comes to behavioral issues.

Right from the start, Sadie refused to sleep anywhere but in Shane's bed. Not on his bed but in it. She loved to burrow about until she became satisfied with just the right pile of blankets covering her body. The relationship appeared to be mutual, for on many occasions I saw Shane wandering through the house at night looking for Sadie because it was "their" bedtime. I remember one night when Shane came running out of his bedroom shouting, "Dad, Sadie has this big growth on her ear! I was petting her in the dark and felt it!" I hurried into his room to inspect her ear, and, sure enough, a thumb-sized growth protruded from it.

I explained to Shane that it was just a wood tick, and I carefully extracted the nasty critter from her ear. We live out in the woods, and I must have missed her monthly application of 'Tick-be-Gone." Some veterinarians can be such lousy examples of the proper care and feeding of pets, but then I know a few pediatricians guilty of the same kinds of lazy neglect.

When I glanced up at Shane, I noticed that he looked as if he were about to vomit. "A tick!" he gasped as he began tearing off his bedding, inspecting every nook and cranny with painstaking care, certain he would find a nest of creepy, crawly, bloodsucking ticks. After completing his lengthy search of the bedding, he turned his attention to Sadie. I know she enjoyed that attention, for it must have felt to her more like a whole body massage than a search. Shane refused to sleep with Sadie that night – the first and only night they were apart. I believe Shane never felt quite as comfortable with his furry friend snuggling up to him in the dark after that night.

I think Sadie would agree that life was good to her. The only exception to her idyllic life as an adolescent was the occasional trip to the groomer. Many clients tell me that as soon as they turn down the road leading to the vet's office, their animal begins to shake uncontrollably. They are convinced that their pet is fully aware that in a few moments he or she will be standing on my exam table with a thermometer sticking out of his or her bum.

Sadie went through a similar experience when I turned down the road leading to the groomer. She despised water (which must have baffled my two retrievers) nearly as much as she hated the sound and feel of clippers. I always felt I had to apologize to the groomer after hearing stories of my pup's unruly behavior. As her groomer described it, "Grooming Sadie is like attempting to get a frightened cat out of a cage. All you can see is teeth, tonsils, and claws!"

To that unholy mix Sadie would add the pungent aroma of freshly discharged anal-gland secretion. I believe this addition to her list of less-than-welcome behaviors was purposeful. It was a way of punishing me for bringing her to the groomer, knowing it would "guilt" me into paying extra! And then I would leave the groomer making the same lame excuse every client has made to me when a pet has been unruly on the exam table: "She's never like that at home, Doc," or "He's never ever bitten anyone before! Sorry, that must really hurt!" I sometimes wonder what goes through Sadie's groomer's mind as she sees my pickup pull up in front of her establishment. On second thought, maybe it's better I don't know.

Our rural setting was idyllic for our canine family, ticks aside. Our home, away from the city traffic, allowed me to give the dogs more freedom than their city-dwelling cousins could claim. Sadie insisted on being included on walks into the woods behind our home in spite of my insistence that the big dogs come along. I'm sure she didn't want me to think that her efforts to keep up with them were an admission that she cared about them.

I remember fondly the summer days when the alfalfa fields grew tall and Sadie had to rise up on her hind legs to keep an eye on the whereabouts of the four-legged family members, then lower herself onto all fours and head off in their general direction, only to stand again to reorient herself to their ever-changing direction. Soon her tongue would stick out, quickly moving back and forth to the rhythm of her pant. She was such a vain little dog, but down deep she loved the adventure of just being out with us.

It was here at our house, among the weeds, where Sadie found her niche: finding and killing rodents. It was the only time she could take on another living creature and win, since she generally challenged opponents far larger than she was. I rewarded her hunting skills by giving her medication to kill the tapeworms she contracted from eating an occasional mouse or two. (I never told Shane I had been treating her for tapeworms. The ear-tumor episode had nearly done him in.)

It was during one of our outings through the fields, when we were passing through some thick underbrush, that Sadie let out a sharp yelp. Startled, I glanced down to see her pawing at her left eye. I quickly reached down and picked her up to try to see what was bothering her. She was squinting her left eye and tears were flowing down onto her muzzle. I had to hold onto her little legs to keep her from attempting to rub at what hurt. I worried she might scratch her eye with one of her nails, which could easily create a much bigger problem.

As I carried her back to the house I could feel her trembling, a sure sign that she was in pain. Before placing her in the truck for our trip to the clinic, I placed a tee shirt over her neck, taping it about her body to trap her legs inside so that she couldn't continue to rub at her face during the trip. I placed her on the floor, fearing she might roll off the seat and further hurt herself. I was worried because little dogs with bulging eyes are at great risk for corneal injury.

When we arrived at my clinic, I administered several drops of a topical anesthetic into Sadie's eye and waited for it to take effect before beginning my exam. I suspected that she might have gotten a grass seed (also called a foxtail or cheat grass) trapped behind her third eyelid. Such seeds are very abrasive and are capable of doing incredible damage if they go undetected. Their favorite hiding place is behind the third eyelid, a delicate membrane you sometimes see covering the eye when a dog is tranquilized or when the eyelid is inflamed.

Using a pair of small forceps, I grasped the numbed third eyelid and pulled it gently forward. And there, down in the cavity between the third eyelid and the cornea, lay the culprit, a "frond" of cheat grass. With my technician firmly holding Sadie, I grasped the cheat grass with a pair of forceps, and out it came from its stubborn hiding place.

After I flushed out the dog's eye with a solution, I applied a fluorescent dye to see if the cornea might take a stain. Normal corneal tissue will not stain. The presence of a stain indicates, in a case like this one, that the cheat grass may have caused an abrasion on the surface of the cornea. Sure enough, there was a very superficial pale area of staining. The cornea is extremely sensitive, so it was no surprise that Sadie had so desperately tried to rub her eye or that it had teared so badly.

I was lucky to have been there at the moment this injury took place, and the fact that I was able to bring Sadie in right away and remove the cheat grass immediately would prevent the more serious injury that would have occurred if the original trauma had been left undetected for any length of time. But still, there was that pale stain. Any time the integrity of the corneal tissue is disturbed, there's a chance of infection. I thought that thoroughly flushing Sadie's wound with an eyewash and putting her on an ophthalmic drop containing an antibiotic should minimize the chances of infection. I felt sure she was going to be all right.

On our way, our little dog lay quietly beside me, drifting along in a world of sedated euphoria. Fastened securely around her neck was the not-so-trendy lampshade. It was Sadie's very first time to don the "e-collar," a necessary precaution to protect her from herself. I wasn't taking any chances with her rubbing her eye. It took several days before she finally gave up trying to dislodge the collar. I think sheer fatigue led her to give in to it. Neither of us had any idea that the hated cone would be with her for a very long time.

Sadie quickly became very adept in the art of walking with an e-collar. I would take her out each day to let her do her business, and she would strut about the yard, head held high, conveying an air of privilege. In truth, her regal posture was necessary to keep her from snagging the lip of her collar in the grass. Her head and collar would sway back and forth, moving her limited view of the world from the few scattered clouds overhead to the tops of nearby pine trees.

Suddenly, she would be overcome with curiosity, perhaps hearing an interesting sound or sniffing a strange smell that would lure her into lowering her head to investigate. Suddenly, the lip of her lampshade would catch on the grass, and, like a pole-vaulter, she would be launched skyward in a perfect forward summersault, landing on all fours like an accomplished canine gymnast. She would nonchalantly shake herself and continue on as if nothing out of the ordinary had just occurred. She repeated this acrobatic maneuver several times during each of our daily outings.

But the eye worsened. The medications I was using to guard against infection failed. I could tell when she began to squint and keep her eye partially closed. When I first noticed her discomfort, I took her back to my clinic and re-stained her cornea. Sure enough, the abrasion had become an ulcer.

Our city is fortunate to have a veterinarian who specializes in eye conditions, so I took her in to see him. Over the next several months, we did everything to get her eye to heal: cultures, medications, surgery to close the eye and protect the cornea, and scraping (debriding) the unhealthy tissue. Finally, the eye began to heal and I again became guardedly optimistic.

Then, several weeks later, I noticed her squinting again. In we went to re-stain her cornea. And there it was, an eerie green glow where the stain clung to the ulcer, an ulcer bigger than before. Things went rapidly from bad to worse after that, leaving us with one remaining option: to remove Sadie's eye. Her eye condition had been as stubborn as her personality, and in the end she lost the battle. Her eye had to be surgically removed.

I thought about how invasive it would be to have an eye removed, and I was fearful that it might go as badly as her ulcer had gone. She had suffered through several months already, and I wasn't looking forward to the surgery at all.

I was preparing for the worst.

I thought about having another veterinarian do the surgery. I know that working on your own pets is not wise. But surgery was my strength, and I had done this particular surgery quite a few times during my long career. I decided to do the surgery myself, and I'm thankful that it went well.

And then a small miracle came along. Sadie's recovery was nothing short of remarkable. She instantly felt better, and it was then that I understood the chronic pain of her eye was greater than I had realized. This was confirmed by how quickly she became a much younger dog! The surgery released her from the bondage of chronic pain. I had new respect for how painful eye diseases can be.

The day I brought Sadie home, we all noticed the remarkable change in her behavior. She ran around the room banging her collar off the walls, scampering about like a puppy. As soon as the stitches were removed, so was her "cone." Her world suddenly got bigger. She was free at last. She once again became our little obnoxious Shih Tzu, our little canine Cyclops.

Sometimes at night, when the light hit her remaining eye at just the right angle, it would glow like a single orb, giving her the appearance of an alien. And she walked with an ever-so-slight head tilt to the side of the missing eye, giving her the appearance of a small dog about to make a left-hand turn. Sometimes she did turn, but mostly she just kept going straight.

When Sadie was eight human years old, she acted as if she were two. Small dogs live longer on the average than the larger breeds, and I was sure she was on track for a long happy life. Lois and I had decided to take a trip up to one of the lakes near our home, and we took Sadie along with us to give our two hunting dogs a reprieve from her incessant need to boss them around. She jumped into her position of entitlement on the console between the front seats of my truck, and I could tell she was excited. Sadie loved riding in my pickup.

A few hours later we reached our destination and parked alongside the shores of Priest Lake, Idaho near the border with Washington State. There is something magical about lakes in the summer when the water warms, when kids and dogs alike play along the shoreline, doing what kids and dogs do best. It was that kind of day, and the lake was calm.

Our plan was to follow a path along the shoreline and let Sadie explore. We knew she would stay away from the water's edge, since her breed is programmed to shun water unless it's in a small bowl for drinking. The Shih Tzu creed is "No swimming, no bathing, no wading."

But Sadie immediately ran down to the water's edge and began drinking. At first I was amused at her sudden show of courage, but as she continued to drink I began to realize something other than courage was at work here. Lois had a puzzled look about her: "I've never seen her go near the water. Have you?" We walked over to where she was busy lapping away. She took no notice of us, and continued drinking. I reached down and picked her up in my arms. Her little body was on fire! She felt hot, very hot, and I was shocked. Just a few hours ago she'd been fine, but now she certainly wasn't. She lay listlessly in my arms, and I knew she was in need of immediate medical attention.

We drove back to Spokane. On our way into town I

decided to go to our emergency animal hospital; it was Sunday, and I knew they would be open. A number of years before, a group of veterinarians, including me, went in together to build an emergency facility for pets in our city. The purpose was to take care of our clients' pets during our off-hours, weekends and holidays, sort of like a pet ER.

Today was my turn to be a client, and I was relieved knowing the clinic would be open and fully staffed to help Sadie. I liked taking care of my own pets for the little things, but when I thought something major was wrong I lost objectivity. I knew it was better to entrust the care of my animals to others especially those who staffed the emergency hospital. It was comforting to have Sadie under their competent care.

Our little dog's temperature was 105.2. She was rapidly weakening, and I feared she would lapse into a coma. They put her on IV fluids and ran blood work. The results came back shortly, and it was clear that Sadie's problem had to do with her kidneys. Her kidney test was off the chart, and her urine was full of bacteria. The rest of her blood work was normal, other than results showing a very high white-cell count, consistent with infection. Antibiotics were added to the IV drip she was already on.

Again, Sadie responded remarkably well. By the next day her temperature was back in the normal range, and she was much more alert. I took her home on oral antibiotics and followed up on a series of blood tests over the next several months. Her kidney test results continued to be slightly higher than normal but much lower than the initial levels. For a while, she seemed better. Shane would be the one who first picked up on subtle signs that she just wasn't herself. It was then that we discovered she was spilling protein into her urine. The presence of protein and the persistent mild elevation in kidney values caused enough concern that I took her in to have an ultrasound performed by a veterinarian who specialized in "imaging"– a person whose skills in this particular area were widely respected by members of our veterinary community.

Sadie's kidneys did not image normally, so the vet performed a kidney biopsy using ultrasound as a guide. With a special biopsy needle and ultrasound, he could obtain a sample from her kidney without putting her through major surgery. The pathology report confirmed that she had a progressive disease that would certainly shorten her life. The pathologist estimated she would not live more than a year or two, at most. Of course we were all upset, and Shane sulked about the house, not wanting to accept the report.

I think it is helpful when veterinarians go through these difficult medical problems with their own pets. It helps us appreciate what our clients go through as they deal with their pets' medical problems, and it gives us a better understanding of their anxieties and fears when the bond with a beloved pet is threatened. I know that it has helped me relate better with my clients when their pets are faced with complicated wounds and diseases.

Staying true to her imperious nature, Sadie made the pathologist look like a fool by far exceeding his two-year prognosis. She wasn't cured. She had her bad times, and on several occasions she had to be placed back on IV fluids. But she always rallied and was able to maintain her elevated position in our family. She continued to bring grief to her groomer, and she never passed up any opportunity to intimidate a Rottweiler, a Great Dane, a pit bull, or a coyote that might stray into her territory. She lived six more years – six good years – following her diagnosis.

I knew the end was coming close when she suddenly began losing weight. The rate of protein loss from her "leaky" kidneys had accelerated, and we were no longer able to keep her healthy through nutrition. The day she refused to take our walk out into the fields was a very sad day. I saw her watching from the window, head slightly turned to favor her remaining eye, as Bailee, Shilo and I headed out for our walk. It broke my heart. A mere week later, she was laid to rest in the presence of her family, including her favored one, a heart-sore and grieving Shane.

Part Two
Vet Stories

Pets & Children

I thought I knew a lot about the bond from my practice and my own family experience, but one day I had my eyes opened even wider when I had the daunting task of talking to a class of eight-year-olds, third-graders, about pets. I have given lots of talks over the years to adults about various pet topics, but this was my first go at the challenge of talking to a room full of two-legged puppies. I was a tad apprehensive.

I stood in front of the room, gazing at the silent youngsters, wondering just how to begin to speak to them. I could read the questioning expressions on their faces and guessed it was going to be like pulling teeth to get them to participate. I dreaded the thought of spending an hour boring these kids with my monologue. I glanced over at the teacher, noticing that she was smiling at me as if to say, "Go ahead – say something, say anything, just get started." I cleared my throat and began: "Who here has a pet?"

My expectation was for a few tentative hands to go up. Perhaps the bravest kid would risk talking to this strange gray-haired adult standing before them. I've never been so wrong in my life. The class erupted with dozens of lively little hands waving madly in the air. The "me first" fest had begun, catching me off balance and unsure about just how to manage such frenetic activity. I felt as if I had just entered a room full of puppies thinking I could bend down and pat just one. I looked over at the teacher again, wondering if she sensed my apprehension, but she had the same smile as before – friendly but unhelpful. I decided to point at the nearest child, and I asked, "What's your pet's name?"

The child answered. Then another piped up. I learned a lot that day. The hour flew by, as the excited children told me all about what made their dogs and cats so lovable, so special. A deluge of colorful animal names was followed by interesting descriptions of shapes, sizes, and colors that danced the time away. They wanted me to know where their pets slept, what they ate, their favorite toys, where and how they pooped.

But mostly they told joyous stories. Stories created whenever pets, like living catalysts, are adopted into human families. These stories arose from the children's deep attachment to their adopted creatures, and they offered clear evidence of the presence of the bond between child and pet.

I was amused when a minor scuffle broke out among several rowdy kids. They argued over who had the better pet – a variation on "Whose dad's the strongest?" I was relieved when the teacher finally did step in to restore order.

Even though I was definitely out of my element, I warmed to the kids' enthusiasm. After a while, their quarreling quieted, giving me the chance to risk another question: "What does your pet need to be happy?" I was curious to find out just what these youngsters might know about the care of pets.

As many hands as before began waving in renewed excitement. I was astounded at how perceptive these small humans were to the needs of their pets. I began writing out their responses on the blackboard. It was an impressive list: pets need food and water, a warm place to sleep, a safe place away from cars; they need to play, they like exercise, they need to go to the vet when they don't feel too good (I liked that one!), they need their shots.

A freckle-faced girl in the back offered, "We took our doggie to doggie school so he'd learn not to jump up on me all the time." Another said, "Sometimes pets need a bath when they stink." A well-groomed boy shouted out, "They need to be brushed so they don't get hairballs!"

But what caught my attention and what I heard over and over again was this: they like to be petted and hugged – a lot.

As I was writing out the children's list of their pets' needs on the blackboard, I had an interesting thought. These third-graders have just created a great handbook covering most of the essential ingredients necessary to raise healthy, happy pets.

Parents who mentor their children in applying this list (at an age-appropriate level of responsibility) would be teaching the basic skills of good pet "parenting." In fact, I think this is exactly what many families already are doing. Pets give parents the opportunity to begin training their kids in the skills they'll need when they have their own children.

Throughout my veterinary career, I have encouraged my clients to bring their children into my office with them. I enjoyed answering questions in the exam room asked by inquisitive kids, and I believe that most veterinarians also enjoy this "family" aspect of our profession.

I was pleased when I heard how many parents took their kids with them to puppy classes and, later, to various animal-training and obedience classes. These are great places for younger family members to learn positive training techniques for their pets, using rewards rather than punishment to accomplish desired behaviors.

At home, many of the tasks outlined in our class "What

Pets Need" list are great opportunities for parents to reinforce in their kids the importance of these responsibilities and why they must be done consistently. I laughed as I recalled some of my clients telling me they actually used techniques learned in pet obedience training on their kids when training them to become good pet "parents!"

I would be remiss to leave out the one task most folks have difficulty with: "poop patrol." This is where children demonstrate incredible skills learned in pet obedience classes – to train their parents by using rewards (the promise of good behavior) in order to escape the dreaded "poop patrol."

At some point, as we help our children become responsible caretakers of their pets, parents become conscious of something I believe they already know intuitively: the bond they have with their children and the bond their children are developing with the family pet forms, in part, around the completion of these tasks.

Children come to realize that "bond" is actually a verb on its way to becoming a noun. This seems most true when kids play with their pets. Here, their two natures blend together in a most natural way, as two different creatures interacting in mutual love of play.

As I listened to the third-graders, I realized that the joy I was seeing came from this same bond, this child-pet bond. I noticed especially how quickly the children's enthusiasm erupted whenever their stories embraced times of play. I got caught up in their contagious excitement.

Their stories contained so many examples of touch – petting, wrestling, hugging, or simply having a kitten curled up in their laps. My counselor's words came to me once again:

"Everyone needs hugs daily. It takes two hugs a day to survive, four to maintain, and six to grow."

He wasn't talking about pets at the time, but I believe not only that what he said is true, but also that some (perhaps many) of those "hugs" do come from pets. For children on the short end of human hugs, a pet can make up for some of the loss. We humans can be touched by a soft-spoken word or an act of kindness, but there is no good substitute for a gentle touch that says "I care."

Pets are spontaneous and generous in their affection for their human siblings, and during times when a parent fails to notice that his or her child needs to be held or touched, the pet is always there. That's a win-win situation, for pets, too, are in need of affection – and families with children are Mecca for pets in search of a playmate – and a hug.

I'm biased when it comes to believing that families are completed when a pet is present. Whether because of the free hugs, the unconditional acceptance of humans, the love of play, or animals' innate ability to bond with us, families benefit from their presence. There is an ineffable quality to our relationship with pets that intrigues me. I sometimes tire of the scientist in me always searching for answers, and it is comforting to relax and let the bond just be, to accept the fact that some things are beyond our complete understanding. I sometimes wonder if whatever it is that brings human and pet together in mutual affection might be somehow spoiled if it were examined too closely. There is something humbling about mystery.

A Vet & His Pets

I've been blessed with having pets almost my whole life.

One of my earliest experiences of the power of the bond came when I was a latchkey child for a year or so when my mother went to work to shore up the family finances. I no longer came home to the sweet, spicy aroma of cinnamon rolls and the warmth of my mother's voice as we chatted about the day at school.

Gone are those pleasant days. I entered an empty house, silent and foreboding. My boyish imagination conjured up intruders and unwanted guests, hiding behind the closet door and under my bed. Hungry, I sat and waited on dark winter afternoons for headlamps coming up the driveway to chase away the fear. By spring there was another change as I opened the door each day. It was the sound of a high-pitched bark coming from somewhere inside, responding to my whistle, hearing my shout, "Here Lassie!"

Then came the clatter of nails clicking against the hardwood floor. Suddenly, my first canine companion would shoot around the corner. Traveling a bit too fast, she would careen into a wooden chair and right herself. I'd scoop her up in my arms as she licked and whined and carried on as though I were a long-lost friend. She was a clumsy pup: a shiny, black Labrador retriever, who grew quickly into her huge paws. I remember feeling the warmth of her shiny fur against my cheek. I was safe, and my house had once more become a home.

In a sense, I was – and am – at home in life when I am with my pets. There were so many times in my youth when another animal, my best and most loyal friend, Hobo, a black-and-white mongrel, was there for me – not only as my constant playmate, but also my "consoler" during times when I was quite sure I was being treated unfairly by my parents for testing their much-too-restrictive rules. I felt that my job as an unruly kid was to push the boundaries as far as possible, and Hobo would always take my side. His love was unconditional.

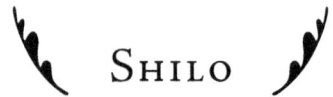 Shilo

Even though I had had decades of professional and personal experience with pets of all kinds, and had a yellow Lab, Abby, I was quite unprepared for the rigors of having canines from two high-energy breeds in the family: Shilo, another yellow Lab, and Bailee, our black-and-white Springer spaniel. They have taken my understanding of, and appreciation for the bond to another level as teachers, companions and inspirations. Even though both joined the family as pups at the same time, Shilo always seemed to come first as she would be first to bolt forward in greeting people in the flesh. And so I'll tell her story first, intertwined as it is with Bailee's.

Strangely, unlike most of her hunter breed, Shilo had absolutely no interest in birds. Like most of her kind, she did have a gluttonous appetite and a tail wag that bordered on dangerous. Her hunting passion, however, took a perverse turn from winged creatures to animal droppings, preferably those of deer.

Her keen sense of smell was enough to locate her preferred prey, which she found in abundance on the floor of the forest near our home. They offered no resistance to being hunted down and devoured, and she consumed them with as much fervor as normal Labs have for bird hunting. Her other delicacy, thankfully less abundant, was rotting animal carcasses. It would be unfair not to credit Shilo with at least a hint of hunting instinct. She did, on rare occasions turn to furiously digging for rodents, who almost always eluded her frantic paws in their maze of tunnels. I suspect living creatures might have offset the stale aftertaste of carrion or deer poop.

Her efforts as a rat catcher were usually so futile that I wondered why she didn't give it up for good. Then, one day on a walk, I saw her launch herself once again into trench warfare with the elusive rodents. She began to wear down, and I suspect she was about to surrender the battle when her head appeared with a rodent firmly secured by its tail between her front teeth. What happened next astounded me. She tossed the struggling vole up into the air, and as it arced back down she caught it in mid-flight and swallowed it whole, bypassing teeth and taste buds in the process. She seemed so pleased with herself, as if that single, un-tasted morsel was sufficient reward for all that digging.

Shilo had that same triumphant air when she sniffed out a fresh sampling of droppings or decomposing flesh; she acted like a kid who has found an unguarded cookie jar. I don't know which was worse after one of her forays: her licking me following a recent "find" or the overpowering stench of her foul breath wafting my way as she sits, panting, upwind of me.

If Shilo wasn't eating smelly things, she was wearing them.

I think of her as a canine Van Gogh who preferred the earthy brown hues of nature's waste to vibrant colors. Her technique was to roll in the fresh, organic pigments, legs skyward, to ensure full coverage on her back, and sometimes wiggle energetically to grind them into her yellow canvas. Regardless of method, the result was more camouflage than art. As with most of Shilo's objectionable behavior, my attempts to discourage her always met with stubborn resistance.

Shilo was a collector as well as an eater and digger. In a single season she had retrieved from the woods a treasure trove of deceased-animal body parts: a selection of deer legs in varying stages of decomposition, several antlers, an entire ribcage, and a skull with one eye still intact. Normal folks have playgrounds with swings and sandboxes full of colorful buckets and plastic shovels. I have body parts in my yard. There is no doubt from those passing that dogs have replaced children at our home. My kids have all grown and moved on, taking with them all signs of human trappings and leaving the entire yard to be filled with organic canine toys.

Labs don't wag their tails. A "wag" implies a gentle, benign, to-and-fro movement of the tail that broadcasts a friendly affection toward the object of the wag. Shilo's tail movement was much too dangerous to be called that. With whip-like speed her tail knocks over small children, sweeps coffee tables clean, and drums against the walls of our house, making a sound like a serious remodeling project in progress.

Over the years I have had clients bring their dogs into my practice with injuries to the tips of their tails because of this kind of "wag." It's baffling that some dogs, mostly hunting breeds, with Labs being overrepresented, wag their tails with such force that they damage the tip.

Picture what the inside of my exam room looks like after one of these "tail-whipper" breeds brings its injury into my clinic.

Each wag sprays blood about the room, covering the walls and humans with a fresh red splatter pattern that suggest a real crime scene.

It's a challenge to heal these wounds because it appears as if the waggers are insensitive to pain and don't mind banging their partially healed tails until the wounds reopen. I have put plastic casts on the tips of dogs' tails to act as a cushion, only to have the casts come flying off like errant missiles. Sometimes as a last resort, I've had to shorten the tail surgically as the only way to stop the bleeding and re-injury. I am thankful Shilo has escaped such a fate. Why her tail has remained sound throughout these years of drumming remains a mystery.

One injured Lab tail remained a mystery until I humbled myself and asked an older colleague for help. Every veterinarian just starting out needs the advice of a seasoned vet such as my friend Clyde to help out on occasion, and this was my occasion. The young Lab arrived at my clinic with his tail hanging limply between his back legs. His guardian said, "I don't know what happened, but his tail hasn't moved since yesterday, not even when he poops!"

I had barely touched the tail at the start of my exam when he let out a sharp cry of pain. I could see no external evidence of trauma, and the X-rays revealed a very normal tail, free of fractures and other abnormalities. I was stumped. I called ol' Clyde, and before I could finish giving him all the information, he was laughing. I asked him what was so funny, and he replied, "It's swimmer's tail. Just ask your client if he has had his pet in the water lately."

My client nodded his head, telling me that, indeed, he had been to the lake two days before. There'd been no problem before the outing. It turns out that swimmer's tail is caused by a dog swimming after a prolonged period of being out of the water. That's why most cases are diagnosed in late spring or early summer.

The theory is that when a dog is swimming, the tail acts as a rudder and is "wagged" differently, and against more resistance, than when the dog is out of water, where the wagging tail is held in a slightly arched position over the back. As a result, during the dog's long-awaited swim, the tail muscles become fatigued, inflamed and painful. The condition is probably similar to our pain when we suddenly overdo our exercise following a New Year's resolution.

The treatment for swimmer's tail is pain medication and rest, and in just a few days the dog will be up and wagging – and pooping – quite normally. Swimmer's tail is one of very few conditions that can successfully overcome the dog's desire to wag.

I believe Shilo was also born with a condition that has a genetic basis to explain her inability to control her activity level. Somehow, she missed the hunting gene for seeking out fowl and instead got a double dose of whatever is responsible for her energy level. Hyper falls short of describing just how over-the-top she is. Were Shilo human, she would probably be diagnosed as unipolar: bipolar without the depression. Pure, high-octane mania. I like to refer to Shilo as "spirited" when we're out in public; it sounds less clinical when I'm apologizing to folks for her disruptive behavior.

There is no way I can get her to be still. Once she had an infected left eye that I had to medicate four times daily. I think I got most of the ointment in the infected eye because she eventually got better. Treating my own pets helped me become a better, more sympathetic doctor when advising clients just how to go about medicating more energetic dogs at home.

Once I finally accepted Shilo "just the way she was," my frustration with her began to wane. My patience grew as I realized it was her immutable nature, her zest for life that I struggled against. I even found myself a bit envious over her carefree approach to life. She never walked, she danced. I wondered if perhaps my "nature" might be frustrating to her? If so she never once let me know. I was accepted – unconditionally.

I must admit that I did try to tame her when she was still a wee pup. In retrospect it was really a very poor decision on my part. I decided I would do what I recommend to all my clients, and I signed her up for what is supposed to be a fun experience: a puppy class, a sort of canine boot camp. I thought that by waiting a few weeks before enrolling her, she might mature and mellow out a bit, and I made the mistake of holding her back.

On the first day of class I noted how much bigger Shilo was than most of the other pups, with the exception of a Great Dane that was sitting obediently at her master's side. Shilo immediately bolted over to greet this lethargic puppy giant, giving my arm a wrenching jerk when she reached the end of the leash. I knew at that moment that we were destined to be the class misfits. I could see it in the eyes of every pet and every human, and especially on the sullen face of the instructor.

Our stint in school was brief. We were summarily discharged from doggy kindergarten at the end of the second session. The instructor, whom I judged to be a disgruntled army drill sergeant, deemed us too disruptive for the other, more serious-minded students. None of the other attendees seemed sad to see us go, either. I could feel their eyes boring into me as I dragged poor Shilo away from all her newfound canine friends. As we were leaving, I overheard some nasty comments. I was especially offended by one lady whispering to the man next to her just loud enough for me to hear, "That dog needs to be on Ritalin."

On our way home I glanced over at Shilo, who was sitting on the passenger seat next to me totally oblivious to what had just happened to us. I was envious at how incapable she was of feeling like a failure, a feeling so devastating to us humans. She looked over at me with an expression that seemed to say, "Lighten up, Bob. It's just another great day in a dog's world!" I reached over and patted her on the head as I resigned myself to the daunting task of homeschooling. She has doggedly (there is no other word) refused ever to surrender her puppyhood. At 12 years, she still doesn't walk; she dances. I have often wondered just what it is between Shilo and me that makes me so helplessly attached to her. Am I addicted to chaos? No, I'm not. But my attachment to this wild-child dog is evidence of the bond at work in spite of the chaos.

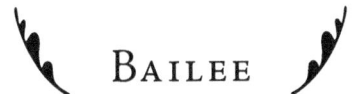

Bailee

Bailee was a welcome contrast to Shilo. Both were spirited, but Bailee had an "off-on" switch to her energy level while Shilo was stuck in the "on" position. Each evening as I climbed out of my truck, both would be waiting for me. At first glance Bailee would appear quite calm until you looked at her stubby tail. Its relative shortness reduces its "drag" and makes the "wag" a blur. It would be a real breakthrough to tap into the energy emitted by my pets' tail wagging and use it to say, power up a generator to run power tools or heat a home in January.

If Shilo was a rogue and a family scapegoat, Bailee, the calm one, was the family hero. She had a disquieting habit of staring. Bailee would sit directly in front of me and look directly into my eyes with an intensity that made me uncomfortable. Maybe the stare makes me feel like she's doting on me, that she wants to be in my presence. Perhaps as a human, I am not accustomed to how it feels to be so unconditionally accepting. Don't I need to do something exceptionally nice to her to deserve such acceptance? Or is it something else? Maybe I give off something I am not aware of that she can sense, a sixth sense that only canines can detect?

I think this thing I've been calling the bond might have to do with things we are not even aware of as people. We humans are supposed to be the sentient members of the human-animal bond, or so we tell ourselves. Is there still a mystery that surrounds our attachment to our pets that science can't explain? I for one hope so because I sincerely believe we have much to learn about our pets, how they communicate, how they detect subtle changes in the emotional states of their guardians. Maybe Bailee was just teasing me, encouraging me to accept that there is great mystery surrounding the essence of our bond.

Petting Bailee had a tranquilizing effect, putting her into a trance-like state. It had the opposite effect on Shilo, triggering her mania from the first stroke of the hand. When both were present, the competition to be the favored one erupted with comical effect; Bailee was immobilized by my touch while Shilo danced in a childlike ecstasy of head bobbing and tail wagging. Only when Shilo got between Bailee and me, did Bailee suddenly awaken from her trance and forcefully shift her body to crowd out Shilo.

Bailee's relative calmness might lead one to suspect that she has a medical condition or is just plain lazy. But these thoughts would vanish were you to see me open the door and step outside. Once Bailee perceived I was headed for a walk, she exploded and instantly attained Shilo-level energy, her hunting instinct fully unleashed. Bailee had the true nose of a bird hunter. That is her passion. I hadn't quite grasped the depth of Bailee's hunting ability until the day I brought her home from her surgery.

True to the biological rhythm of her species, Bailee was nearing that wonderful time in her life when her reproductive clock would strike "period" and push her abruptly out of her brief but cute stage of prepubescent innocence into "HEAT," that seductive condition seemingly capable of drawing male canines out of thin air.

Having a dog in heat introduces you to the potency of the fertility scent. If one tiny molecule of "heat scent" escapes and is blown afar by a gentle breeze, you will experience a sudden explosion of four-legged male visitors who show up on your doorstep and busy themselves with their task of asserting property rights. They resist all efforts to rid yourself of them. They are yours for the duration of your dog's heat – up to three or more weeks!

I didn't want urine markings around the perimeter of my home to be the first indicator that I had waited too long before spaying Bailee. All those years of medical training makes it difficult for some vets to use "spay" as a stand-in for its flashy latinized brethren, ovariohysterectomy. It seems that for some veterinarians the latter helps to justify the cost of the procedure, although the end result is the same whichever word is used: a sterile pet.

On a serious note, I try to avoid using medical jargon carelessly. I once told a client that her pet had a "fatty tumor," a totally benign diagnosis. Her sudden burst of tears caught me completely off guard. I asked her what had upset her. She sobbed out a reply. "When I was a young girl my folks had to have our golden retriever put down because she had a "tumor."

I calmly explained in the simplest terms why the word tumor is not always the same as cancer, as was true in this case. This is an everyday example of how "doctor talk" can unwittingly bring a pet's worried guardian into our medical world, where we feel comfortable. I know I have been careless with jargon many times in the mistaken belief that my medical world is also a comfortable place for folks who are worried about the beloved pets.

Back to Bailee's then impending spaying. One fine spring morning I loaded my unsuspecting virgin into my truck for a trip to the hospital. She seemed so happy sitting by my side, looking out the truck window without the slightest suspicion she was about to be betrayed. How deep that trust runs in the bond.

I spayed her that same morning, before she could sully our good reputation by becoming the seductive neighborhood "bitch in heat." I wasn't going to become like the many clients through the years who looked me in the face and said, "I can't believe she's pregnant, doc. I only let her out once, and she was only out for several hours!"

They soon return, embarrassed, with a box of six to eight mongrel puppies. Then they would invariably ask, "Say, doc, what breed do you think the father was?" I look at the pups and guess. "I think your purebred German Shorthair was mated with a Dachshund. That's why they have those stubby curved legs and the distance from the front legs to the back legs is twice the normal." They look crestfallen as they peer into the cardboard box full of bizarre-looking puppies.

I try to raise their spirits by reminding them that there are as many bizarre-looking humans as there are dogs, so they should be able to find good homes for the puppies. As they leave, I remind them that perhaps they might want to spay their gal before the next heat cycle hits. Because I'd been through this with so many clients, this weird-looking-puppy scenario was not going to happen to me! I did not tell anyone that my cat had kittens because of my nagging habit of procrastination. That I kept secret. After all, I am a veterinarian, and I should know about these things.

Bailee's surgery went very well; I was relieved to have spayed her in time. She awoke from the anesthetic and quickly passed into a fog of painless sedation. I carefully slipped the dreaded cone over her head, securing it firmly about her neck. Veterinarians try to dignify this medieval piece of equipment by naming it an Elizabethan collar rather than by using the more contemporary term: the collar of shame. Bailee came to despise it, but for the moment her altered state had her oblivious.

I have placed this device over many a pet's head to protect them from themselves, but I am unsure who is really most troubled by its presence – the pet or the guardian. My canine patients are endlessly inventive when trying to separate themselves from their cones.

Most dogs try to pull it off by placing both front paws behind the cone near its base and pulling forward with savage ferocity. They will repeat this maneuver until they either realize its futility or they are successful. If they're successful, the owner must then carefully notch the collar slightly tighter, but not so tight as to strangle the poor creature. The guardian must then stand back and hope that this will work.

Another technique involves banging it against objects like small children, coffee tables, and other breakable items in an attempt to kill the collar. This method has met with some success in that it can completely destroy the collar, especially by the larger breeds. The smaller breeds tend to prefer to back out of the collar. Some clients find a perverse humor in this method, as the poor creature looks like some kind of furry windup toy, scurrying randomly about the room in reverse, changing direction at each impact until finally giving up.

Finally, some folks call the vet requesting a sedative and are reminded that their pet is usually already on a pain sedative. They then try to cajole the vet into letting them raise the dosage. This usually ends with the vet saying, "Changing Maggie's dose will not stop the behavior. It will only set it into slow motion."

The best solution is to allow pets to go through all these antics until they exhaust themselves and give up. Veterinarians are frustrated by a particular condition of the guardian that results in the collar coming off: co-dependence. Pets are surprisingly clever at learning how to get their doting humans to do what they want, in this case removing the cursed collar.

The pet, freed from bondage, turns its attention to the sutures. The next day both pet and guardian are back in my clinic to have those sutures replaced. I then must listen to all the reasons the co-dependent human has to shift the blame to me. Most people, including pet lovers, have a very difficult time accepting fault. They hide their embarrassment under anger when they learn that there's a fee to have the sutures or staples replaced. But they do leave the clinic with renewed determination not to cave in to their whimpering pets' demands and to leave the collar on all the time.

Shilo had a surprising reaction to the cone following her spay. She accepted it with little distress and no attempt to remove it! In fact I think she thought it made her special by the way she strutted about the house with great agility, given the handicap of tunnel vision.

My work at the clinic was finished for the day, I carried my now-sterile companion to my truck for our trip home. She slouched next to me on the passenger side; staring but not seeing, drool dangled from her protruding tongue, trapped in a narcotic fog. She was stuck inside her cone, and for the moment her world was surreal.

I ignored the curious stares of children in the car next to us, pointing, laughing, waving, as I waited for a light to turn green. Bailee didn't seem to care about anything. A thought entered my mind: she hadn't urinated all day. My truck still had that new smell to it and I worried the rest of the way home.

Finally we got home. I went around to Bailee's side of the truck and opened the door. Before I could react, she bolted from the truck, banging her lampshade sharply against my arm, landing upright, and quickly escaping my grasp. She was already a step ahead of me, moving quickly, heading for the woods beyond the yard. I could not believe this was happening. She seemed so unconscious during the trip home.

Even with the lampshade affixed to her head, pain medication aboard, and the surgery just six hours old, she outwitted me. I suddenly envisioned her suture line busting open, exposing her tender belly. She was moving quickly, but to the discerning eye her line of travel was a bit random, her stride had deteriorated, going from graceful to awkward, and more loopy and serpentine as she continued to weave her way toward the woods. Charging into the dense underbrush, she disappeared; I could hear her collar as it banged and crashed against anything that obstructed her frenzied progress.

I feared that she might be in a state of terror brought on by her inability to make sense of her distorted perceptions and worried that she would injure herself as she plunged helplessly through the woods. These thoughts raced through my head as I ran after her. Then, suddenly, unexpectedly, and unbelievably a pheasant flew straight out through the trees, madly calling out, passing directly over my head.

Bailee burst through the brush in hot pursuit, her funnel stuffed full of forest trappings—twigs, leaves, moss and dirt. Only a wet black nose poked out from the nest of organic debris that filled her lampshade. She abruptly pulled up next to me, shook her head and spilled her forest collection upon the ground. Bailee looked up at me as if to say, "Did you see that pheasant I flushed?" She seemed so damned proud of herself. I rolled her over to inspect the incision: somehow still miraculously intact. I let out a long deep sigh.

It was then that I realized just how deeply encoded was her instinct to hunt. Her desire to flush game birds was nothing short of what we humans call passion. I can only appreciate this passion vicariously as it so far exceeds my own meager attempts to muster up anything remotely resembling her sublime fervor to hunt. It is this vicarious nature in our relationship, this contagious enthusiasm for life that attracts and bonds me to my pets.

When I experience their passion for life, I become more alive myself. That is why I sometimes overlook their unruly behavior and forgive them, for it is in their nature to explore their world with zest, a zest that beckons me to join them. I think that I give in too easily to my humanness. It's too difficult for me to let loose the stored passion of my childhood, during which I, too, lived an "unruly" life.

I know I cannot fully reach nor sustain the same measure of eagerness as my hunters, but they awaken in me the desire to do so. I know I am my own worst enemy, choosing too often the path that only entangles me in the complexities of life while denying me the joy and vitality offered by simply living in the present. I believe there are many ways to kindle this desire to feel more alive, but for me a simple walk with my pets has always been sufficient. This is why I take time out with my pets – to watch them dance.

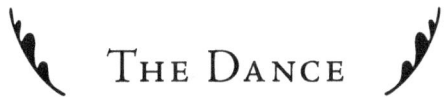 The Dance

Bailee and Shilo lived in the moment with such contagious enthusiasm that it was impossible for me to resist being drawn along with them. They resurrected my memories of bygone times when I, too, could lose myself in the moment and of a place where past and future are swept away as easily as dry leaves scattered by an autumn breeze. The only thing left was a welcomed place of calm I could claim as my own, a place where I feel most alive. Bailee and Shilo's unconstrained zest for life lured me away from the heaviness of my human world; they let me escape from my imagined self-importance.

My pets helped me quiet the busyness of my day; they kept me from ruminating too much on thoughts outside the moment, thoughts of yesterday and tomorrow. When I followed the lead of my two young hunters as they entered the woods and fields surrounding our home, when I entered into the simplicity of their play, my thoughts fell away, surrendering to the moment, into what I have come to call "the dance."

The dance was stamped into their nature as deeply

as instinct itself. The genetic code for the dance trumped other drives in their lives, save that of food. Only food had the power to interrupt their love affair with play. Food and play vied for dominance, throwing my mutts into a state of confusion until one or the other was satisfied. Once one drive was satisfied, the brain instantly switched to the other. That's just the way it works for them. Unfortunately, when "wolfing" down their food – it's by far the most accurate term for their eating style – came first, it was followed by enforced rest. To my pets, that was the same kind of torture my kids endured when we forbade swimming until their food digested. Pets and kids have a natural intolerance for postponing play; obviously the only way to avoid the conflict is to feed after play. It took only one time of enforced rest to convince me to reverse the order.

Days that I feel drained physically and emotionally occur more often as I age (I am 66 as I write). I drag home my work from the clinic, my thoughts pulling me back into the exam room where I let the elderly lady know her elderly cat was nearing the end of its life, or back to a difficult surgery fraught with complications. As I head home, I long for a soft chair in front of the TV, a place in which to just vegetate. I called this little slice of the evening my drool time.

These are the times I hoped my four-legged friends would not be waiting for me when I turned off the main road onto the lane leading home. Alas, I would see them, tails moving wildly as they caught sight or sound of my truck. They knew me and how quickly I'd succumb to their request to dance in their playground: the woods.

Oh, I tried to resist. Sometimes, I went directly inside the house and quickly closed the door before they could wriggle between my legs and enter ahead of me. To get inside ahead of them, before either or both can outwit, out-dodge, or out-maneuver me, requires immense athletic prowess. I feel free to brag about this success only because I've had so many frustrating failures. But why kid myself?

Shutting the door in their faces was the ultimate act of futility. Though I might have won the battle, I lost the war. The battle was not the scuffle at the door but the one in my mind. As I collapsed in the soft chair in front of the TV, the brief thrill of victory was replaced by creeping guilt. I stewed in my thoughts of them outside the door. I saw them sadly waiting, tails wagging, staring at the door, hoping I will give in and join them for our walk. Once again, those two rogues had stolen my mind. I would rise from my chair, turn off the TV, pull on my hiking boots, grab my coat and head for the door.

Once outside the dance began again: Shilo and Bailee have stored enough energy during the day that they are about to explode. They are leaving nothing to chance to entice me, combining their energies in a frenzy of acrobatic leaps, aerial twists and mid-air collisions. If that display fails to capture my attention, Shilo does her solo, a unique running style in which her hind legs overtake her front legs, causing her spine to look like a hunchbacked fur ball careening to devastating comic effect. This burlesque is accented by their jangle of yips, yipes, and yaps that are absolutely disrespectful of the regal behavior expected from such blue-blood breeds. Their routine garners few points for artistic style, but it has proven to be highly successful in winning me over.

Have you ever heard a man or woman you know to be

of a rather serious nature, perhaps even stuffy, erupt into a nonsensical, childish language of baby talk when his or her beloved pet offers a frenzied greeting? This cryptic babble is reserved for the pet's ears only; just the thought of being overheard by other people is mortifying. It is as if pets have the power to suspend the critical messages we give ourselves as to what is adult behavior and what is simple foolishness.

Children also have this mysterious power to release us from our stuffy adult boundaries. Our pets give us permission to cast aside, if just for a moment, the responsible etiquette of adulthood, giving us the green light to enter into foolishness, free of embarrassment. This reprieve requires nothing more than the presence of a pet.

I sometimes think I have become too rigid in my ways. Hardened by the formality of an adult world, I am conditioned to dismiss play as childish, as if it were an activity for youth only. I am thankful for my animal friends, for they help me resist this insidious process of becoming adultified. For me, the only antidote has four legs.

Something wonderful happens when my pets win me over and I enter their world of play. My overly serious side loosens up, allowing fragments of my childhood memories of play to emerge. I find myself longing for that free spirit, the very spirit alive in the play of my pets. They seem to say, "Come down to our level and cavort a bit; leave behind your stuffy rules, and let us resurrect your childlike nature." Have you noticed how many of the "America's Funniest Home Video" clips are of adults being childlike with a pet! I admit that I use my dogs as an excuse to play so I won't be seen as foolish. It is as if pets legitimize adult play.

Once the choreography is complete, we are ready to explore the woods. Both dogs are free to roam on their own, but they choose not to enter the forest without my presence. When I take just a single step in the direction of our woods, they burst ahead as if they have been released from an invisible tether. In the woods, play surrenders to the hunt.

I am mesmerized by Bailee and Shilo moving among the trees with effortless grace, as if gravity has loosened its grip so they glide along the forest floor on lightened feet, guided by a special sense as they dodge bushes and rocks.

This spring day is nature's gift, hard earned during the gray, cold days of winter. The wind is gentle and warm, rich with the scent of fresh pine and lively chatter of birds in the boughs. It lifts a red-tailed hawk on motionless wings to great heights, and then, with a small, almost imperceptible shift of feathers, the hawk alters its path in search of unwary prey: perhaps a rodent scampering along its tiny trail through a nearby alfalfa field.

The green spring grass has grown tall and supple, bending and swaying at the whim of the wind to form graceful patterns across the field. The grass swiftly swallows my hunters; only bending tassels betray their sudden twists and turns. Suddenly, I glimpse Bailee, a blur leaping high above the grass, catching her bearings, disappearing and then resurfacing with only her ears above the blades, lifted by the sheer energy of her gait.

The intensity of Bailee's eyes when she catches sight of a pheasant's sudden flight or the electric quiver of anticipation through Shilo's body just before I release a stick for her to retrieve make the dross of a hectic day drop away. I get swept up in their moment as the wind whispers through pine boughs in the late afternoon light. But they seem unaware of my presence, riveted to the smells and movements about them. Shilo, nose to the ground, searches erratically as some new scents pull her sharply from one direction to another. Bailee cares only for the scent of birds. She lives to flush them from their hiding places and watch them take to the sky. I doubt she feels incomplete in this sport without the crack of a gunshot and a bird to retrieve.

I feel our bond most acutely in these moments, as if some force is orchestrating our dance, weaving together human and animal. The natural harmony of this place has kindled my senses, sweeping aside the noise of my day, offering me a serenity that can be found only in the moment.

I like to play a game that casts this bond in sharp relief, creating a window in time that crystallizes our connection in the moment. It happens when I move quietly from the dogs' sight. From my hiding place, I see them suddenly freeze in their tracks. They are aware that I have disappeared.

Whatever scent or sight occupied their attention just moments before has been pushed aside. They stand motionless, as if deciding what to do next. The dance has abruptly ended. My presence is a necessary ingredient for their game of exploration to work, for the dance to continue. Then they begin an urgent nose-to-ground tracking pattern to pick up my scent. I confess that I have never won this game of hide-and-seek, yet I never tire of it. Shilo, a little slower than her companion, takes longer to find me. When she does, she finds Bailee sitting beside me, looking at her as if to ask, "What took you so long?"

As soon as they find me, they pick up the threads they had dropped moments ago, turn away and redirect full attention to the smells and sounds and sights of the woods. I smile, thinking how strange I would look if someone were to see me, this gray-haired man, running recklessly through the woods, darting behind a tree, crouching motionless, watching my pets yet hidden from their view.

But then, do I really care? I am an adult at play. It's during times like these the differences between pet and human blur. I, too, need the dogs' presence to fully enjoy the dance; I need to feel their presence and watch them move through the shadows of brush, rock and tree. I feel more alive being with them here in the woods. And I savor the mystery in this bond whose invisible tendrils reach out from me to them, from them to me, always bringing us back together in the dance.

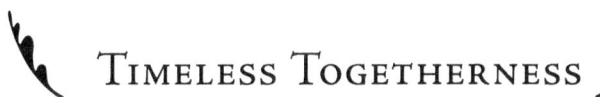

Timeless Togetherness

My four-legged companions have made my life better by helping me with what we humans call time. I have spent a good deal of my life unconscious of its passage. Time moved silently along, unnoticed as I lived through life's stages – college, veterinary school, career, marriage, parenting and grandparenting. It is invisibly embedded in the "doing" of life.

My pets helped me "see" time. Time was made visible by pushing them through life much too fast, leaving in its trail the telltale evidence of its passing – aging. As I watched them age, I became more conscious of my own growing older. The contrast between our biological clocks would bring my awareness of time to the fore. I found myself wishing dogs' time on the planet ran closer to my own.

Seeing time pass through Bailee and Shilo brought with it an unexpected gift: They made time more precious. My dogs helped me understand more deeply that our time is limited – that I had only so much time to be with my two companions. But even if my awareness of its limited nature made time more valuable, more precious, it didn't make my life better. To make this happen, I had to learn a better way to value time. Again, my pets became my teachers.

We humans are not immune to the dark side of aging, knowing time is moving us slowly yet steadily into a state of disrepair. I don't enjoy noticing the symptoms of my advancing age, and it was during a time of stewing over my powerlessness in such matters that my pets came to my aid. It was if they said, "If you can't control time, then maybe you need to consider a better way of spending it."

It was during one of our many walks together in the woods near our home that my lesson began. Here in the forest and the surrounding fields, I began to notice how completely caught up in the moment Shilo and Bailee were. That led me to reflect on how often I ruminate over yesterday's trivial matters or worry about what tomorrow may bring only to miss what is happening in the moment. I realized that I was doing a damned poor job of living in the present.

I sometimes think pets are sent to us from some far off land where time is lived differently. Their mission is to teach humans how to spend our limited time more wisely. The number of clocks we have could be a dead giveaway of our preoccupation with time. But the pets would be sorely pressed to understand why, if we're so concerned about time's passing, do we spend so much of it "outside of time" – in the past or future?

I enjoy wondering what goes on in the minds of my pets, well aware of the dangerous arrogance of pretending that I can know what's happening in there. But I see no harm in imagining what goes on in a dog's or a cat's mind. It is the not knowing that intrigues me, that fires my imagination with curiosity about what inspires my two hunters during our daily walks, especially since they do so completely in the moment.

I believe Shilo and Bailee knew of no other place to be but in the present. If I were to ask them about yesterday or tomorrow, what would they say? Perhaps they would be annoyed and chide me for again falling prey to my obsessive concern over living "outside of time."

They, however, pass from moment to moment, entering each fragment of time fully alert to their world, living life to the fullest. This purity of unencumbered presence must be very freeing. And when I became aware of theirs, I, too, felt the freedom of living within the moment.

I imagine them composing their own living song, a Song of Life, from moment to moment. The lyrics I could not know. They are part of the grand mystery that belongs only to them. But I could witness the music to their song. I "hear" their music in the notes they forge out of each moment of time, each moment an empty vessel of time waiting to be filled with life, to become a part of the song.

These notes are ephemeral by nature and if their passing goes unnoticed, unfilled, they are lost forever. To live this way, living inside each note, moving through life one note at a time, until the last note arrives, is to live life very well indeed. It is wonderfully ironic that by witnessing them create the notes of their song, I am composing my own.

When my two hunters moved through the forest on our walks together I experienced their song as a dance. They were so agile and alive as they moved from note to note, unburdened by past and future as they lived out their song. It is through my bond with them that I sensed this gift they had of living out their song. They had to be patient with me – I am a slow learner about this living in the moment. I am mired in my humanness, and I forsake the moment for careless reasons, over unnecessary distractions.

That ability to be in the moment seemed to give my pets endless enthusiasm and bursts of boundless energy to live life more fully. There is something precious, almost sacred about it, and I felt caught up and swept along with them. Bailee and Shilo became temptresses of time, drawing me in, showing me a better way to "be" in time. They showed me when I strayed from the now and reminded me to return.

When I'm at my best in being in the moment, I experience that intense bond with my pets. I feel a bit foolish admitting that I need my pets' help to realize that a connection to another – whether a pet or a human – must be experienced in the present. I regret how often I have been with people I care about and have allowed living outside of time to disconnect me from them.

If I were to remove from my life all the wasted time spent outside the moment, would I find my pets have actually outlived me? Or perhaps we as humans have been granted more time just so we can learn what our pets know as surely as a bird knows how to build its nest. I think that learning to emulate their gift of living inside each moment is a worthy endeavor. And I will need to turn to them for help when I find myself once again stuck outside of time, stuck in some wasteland of past mistakes or fearful of what tomorrow may bring.

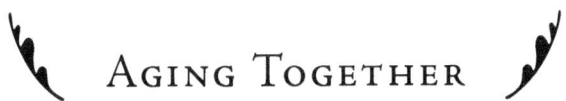 Aging Together

I became aware of the change during one of our walks. I found myself caught up in the moment on a crisp afternoon, when scattered clouds dusted the horizon and the morning chill had lingered under a weak sun. The aspen leaves had begun to turn from pale green to tawny brown and rustled in the breeze. Fall seemed to have descended without notice – as did the sudden realization: my pets had aged.

The impact stopped me in my tracks. How did those gradual changes slip by without me noticing? Had I fallen back into living outside of time, being too busy to see the important things? Or had I shielded myself from unsettling thoughts?

Wasn't I, a veterinarian, trained to notice the subtle changes? It seemed like only yesterday that I'd thought there could be no end to their boundless energy. I even remember wondering if they would ever outrun their frenetic youthfulness to become manageable adults? (Now, that's a true oxymoron: a manageable Labrador retriever). Suddenly it seemed time had sped up and overtaken them, hustling them into the autumn of their lives. I began taking stock of the changes.

Shilo's graceful gait had stiffened; she ran more like a wooden rocking horse than like a wild young pup. Sometimes she stumbled making quick turns. There was a morning stiffness as both dogs rose from their beds to go outside. Shilo ranges closer to me now, and her breathing becomes more labored with less effort. There is more gray in her coat, as well as in Bailee's. How had I failed to notice these things? And when did that graying begin? Did Shilo's yellow coat camouflage the change? When I had Bailee groomed, I was taken aback by the gray hidden beneath her winter coat. I'm sure it wasn't there a year ago.

My reluctance to notice these signs of aging has something to do with our bond. My attachment makes me resist noticing these changes that herald the admission of what I know inside: our time together is limited, and that it's slipping away. It somehow feels like an act of betrayal to acknowledge this thought – as if the act of acknowledging could somehow hasten the outcome. I now understand more fully why many of my clients seem so oblivious to their pets' aging. Like me, they find that they have unwittingly softened reality. "Doc," they would say, "Why is she so …?" There would follow a litany of signs, all relating to the wear and tear of time. I would reply, not unkindly, "Because she's getting older." And they would nod in measured agreement. And here I was, following right along in their footsteps with reluctant nods of my own.

It isn't unusual for my older clients (including me) to become sensitized to our aging pet's infirmities, especially those that seem to mirror our own. When denial no longer obscures our vision, we begin to notice the smaller changes,

changes that would have gone unnoticed earlier.

We are fearful that something more insidious might lie beneath that morning cough, or that water bowl that needs filling more often, or that bit of food left uneaten. We notice these things, and sometimes all we can say is, "She's not quite right. I can't put my finger on it."

We are becoming conscious of the wily nature of aging, which brings with it ailments that often have no cures, and we find ourselves adjusting to a new world of chronic syndromes. Many of them bear the confusing title of "idiopathic." This term appeals to the predilection of the medical community to obscure the truth: we really don't know the exact nature of many chronic disorders. As a colleague once said, "'Idiopathic' means that we are sometimes pathetic idiots."

I enjoyed working with my older clients. I am comfortable with the turn in our conversation as the client begins to realize that a beloved pet's better years are now behind him or her. I remembered when their pets were puppies and kittens. My medical records document the animals' journeys through time, leading up to this older, chronic station in life. I hear both humor and sadness as my clients accept the slow decline of an aging pet just as they accept it in themselves. They – we – are aging as a team, and I think we find comfort in sharing our illnesses with them.

"Doc, that pill you put Shep on is the same darn water pill my doc put me on. We take them at the same time, and, sure enough, we both pee up a storm a half hour later."

"Sadie is drinking and peeing all the time now, and her appetite is huge. She's acting just like me when I was told I had diabetes." And he was right.

"Shep can't hear worth a damn. He used to be a darn good watchdog. Now my wife is telling me to quit worrying about the damned dog and go get myself some hearing aids. I just make her mad by saying, 'What'?" And he laughs.

"I knew you would bring up her weight again. If it isn't my doctor telling me to stop eating anything that tastes good, it's my vet telling me to cut down on Marty's groceries." I don't say anything, noticing they're both overweight. Human and animal doctors share a common bond of impotence when it comes to convincing some humans to shed a few pounds, whether on their own frames or on those of their pets.

"I just had cataract surgery, and I was wondering if you could do the same surgery for my ol' mutt? She used to catch treats, but now she only catches air. But she sure can smell… just turn her loose in the kitchen and you won't find a crumb that survives!"

Very often I hear, "My girl is having trouble getting up in the morning. We both gimp around like old farts. Guess we are. If she feels as bad as I do on some days, I think she should get something to ease the pain a bit." And we discuss ways to manage her pain. And then there's this type of request: "Say, doc, I was wondering if you could put this letter in her medical records? It's about what I want done with her if I pass before she does. I worry about her sometimes, and I'd feel better knowing you know my wishes."

The stories are endless, and they come back to me often, as my dogs remind me that we too have become old farts. I see myself in these stories of aging, and my pets begin to take on the characteristics of many of the pets I have seen over my years of practice. In a way it's like coming home: I imagine all these old folks holding out their hands to me, saying, "It ain't that bad, Doc. All that advice you gave us helped, and now all you have to do is follow along the same trail."

I am more empathetic toward my senior pets when fatigue begins to nag me, reminding me of my own senior status. I often pretend my fatigue is brought on by an unusually hectic day rather than by advancing years. And sometimes it works. I let denial offer me its temporary pardon from reality. Deep down I know that, like the glacier, I will soon be "calving" into retirement.

In times like these, I reach for my antidote. My faithful ally is curiosity: my energy source through all these years remains un-aged and follows me from one exam room to the next, day after day, until decades have passed. Caffeine gets me through the mornings, but it's curiosity that gets me through the day. It turns the most ordinary office visit into something interesting, something to be enthusiastic about.

Veterinary medicine, like human medicine, is constantly changing as a result of an overwhelming influx of new discoveries. Continuing education is not an option. It is a necessity for the vet to stay abreast of new developments. Sometimes, new knowledge renders obsolete what was once taken as gospel. I find it especially worrisome to discover new information that reveals old ways as actually harmful rather than helpful. And so I hear my journals barking for attention, I go to continuing ed classes, and I pick the brains of my fellow vets. Researchers have absolutely no sympathy for the burden they place upon us out here in the field. But there is no doubt – the complexities of my profession are growing, and maybe this is the real source of my fatigue today.

I admit it's not easy to keep up with all the progress our profession has been making over the last 20 years. Specialization has brought with it an increase in board certified veterinarians, doctors on the cutting edge of discoveries and therefore more likely to diagnose and treat conditions that only yesteryear were either still mysteries, untreatable or poorly treated. With their expertise comes new technology such as MRIs, CAT scans, Doppler ultrasound, digital radiology and endoscopy (examining the digestive tract using a camera and light attached to a tube and viewing the pictures on a TV monitor).

While all of this elevates the quality of medicine, it also raises the cost. I am not complaining, I am grateful when I can refer a pet that is in dire need of their help, but I do lament surrendering my antiquated notion that even those folks on limited income should be able to afford a pet and a ticket to a professional baseball game.

Digressing as I just have may be another indication of aging. The mind has covered so much ground over the years and has more experience of life. And how differently aging comes to us all. That is another piece to the story of why we can be caught off guard by the apparent suddenness of our pets' aging. It has to do with the fact that our biological clocks are not synchronized. As different species, they age at different rates. Small-breed dogs (and cats) age more slowly, and giant-breed dogs age more quickly. Bailee and Shilo are large-breed dogs, so I will use their aging rate.

My pets both turned 24 (in human years) when they turned two. Dogs mature rapidly during their first two years, and then slow down to about six human years to each dog year thereafter. By this formula, they turn 60 in dog years when they turn eight in human years. So at eight they are entering what we would call old age.

Here is where my delusion begins. My two hunters turned eight (60 human years) at the very same time I turned 60, yet they neither looked nor acted like seniors (I couldn't say the same about myself!). On our trips into the woods I did not notice any signs of aging. They seemed to run just as gracefully and tirelessly as they had years earlier. Their movements were crisp, eyes alert, ears attuned to sounds beyond the human ear.

Bailee could smell a pheasant at great distances, and Shilo was equally proficient at uncovering the latest deposit of animal droppings. I could detect no decline in them at all; they seemed physically and mentally the same. The fact that their behavior gave no warning signs of their aging had lulled me into believing that they were not like other dogs. No, somehow they had escaped their own biological clocks and had found refuge in my human life-timer.

I had no visible evidence to dissuade me from my delusion, and therefore I was not prepared for the sudden turn in their health over the next two years when they suddenly leapfrogged past me; as I went from 60 to 62, they went from 60 to 72! Suddenly they became old at 10. And that's when I just as suddenly noticed the changes in energy and coat, and the stiffness in gait.

I believe this is what happens to many of my clients' pets when they make their own leap into old age. They suddenly begin experiencing some of the trappings of aging: arthritis, accelerated weight gain, cataracts, indigestion, hearing impairment and low energy, etc. And as pets age, veterinarians begin diagnosing greater numbers with cancer, diabetes, heart problems, kidney disease, skin tumors, lameness and a host of other maladies.

I want to prepare my clients for this sudden progression of age-related health concerns by using my own pets as an example. I caution you not to be skeptical when your veterinarian suggests seeing your pet twice yearly after your animals become seniors! Remember, one year in human time is anywhere from four to ten years – the range from small breeds to that of the giant breeds – in dog time. So taking them to see your veterinarian every six months is really taking them every two to five years in dog time. A lot can happen health-wise in a two to five-year period in our human years. The same is true for our pets.

There is cause for optimism, though, if guardians follow some very simple, sound principles that I have time-tested throughout my career. When we follow these principles our four-legged companions benefit. So do we.

There is no magic involved, no secret elixir or gene therapy – just the practice of three principles: weight control, exercise and staying mentally active. If you and your pet practice these three principles, your physician and veterinarian will suffer a decline in income. Simple, however, is not always easy.

I write this as a challenge to you and your pet to refuse to accept aging passively. If you take up this challenge, you will delay the onset or at least lessen the symptoms of many of the chronic conditions mentioned earlier.

My pets were well into their nineties – and were doing rather well as I wrote most of this book. You could say it's because of good genes, the luck of the draw, and the alignment of the planets. And to a degree you would be right. But since we can't do a heck of a lot with genes and luck (and planets), I would like to focus on the three principles.

First, I worked hard to keep my two companions trim. This is crucial, because both Shilo and Bailee have arthritis. Bailee was born with a condition called hip dysplasia, which predisposed her to degenerative joint disease and arthritis. She has been blessed, for reasons I do not understand, to have remained symptom-free until just a couple of years ago. That's when I noticed minimal signs of weakness and lameness in her hindquarters.

Equally difficult is convincing some clients to readjust their idea of what "trim" looks like. They believe that their pets look svelte, when, in reality, the animals are sometimes markedly overweight. This is especially true when the two-leggeds are also overweight.

Trim is only half of the equation necessary for weight control. The other half is "fit." Shilo, Bailee, and I have taken our walks into the fields and forest surrounding my home since their puppyhood. I am fortunate to have this space because they can be safely off lead, and this freedom allows them to roam at will. I can't say accurately just how much farther they travel on our walks than I do, but let's just say it's substantial – like miles more! As they've aged, they've began to pull back on how far they range, and I try not to overdo our walks.

The reason for pulling back is that many pets, when with their guardians, push themselves beyond what they would normally do. This seems especially true of the hunting breeds, and I caution my clients who hunt to cut back on the time they spend bird hunting as their pets age, because the hunting breeds don't seem to be able to listen to what their bodies are saying, and they will sometimes push themselves to exhaustion.

I don't know whether it's their instinct to hunt or the desire to please their human partners that drives them. I suspect both. I have treated these hunting warriors for heat stroke and acute muscle and/or joint pain because they pushed themselves beyond their waning endurance. I think that what is lacking is common sense on the part of us two-leggeds as we attempt to adapt to the age-related changes that now bedevil our old pets.

When I have ventured too far on our walks, my pets and I are sore the next day. I remember this for our next outing and attend to the delicate balance between enough and too much. It's yet another type of caring, one that requires greater compassion and deeper love on my part. To deny them walks would certainly hasten the weakening of muscle tone and the stiffening of joints, a syndrome familiar to the two-legged as well. I recently began adding dietary supplements to my dogs' diets and using some of the newer pain medications and have been pleasantly surprised at how they have responded. I believe they are doing better than most of their "peers," and I think they know this, too. Sometimes I imagine there's a bit of a swagger in their gait. I can no longer say that they are willowy, or graceful in their movement, but at their age an old-dog swagger is as good as it's going to get.

Finally, I believe that pets are susceptible to the disease of boredom. I call it a disease because if not addressed I believe it causes a more rapid decline in animals' health, especially their mental health. Like us, pets, can experience mental decline. We humans are encouraged to keep our minds active, to remain curious about life. Feline literature refers to keeping cats engaged in life as "environmental enrichment." I call it a walk in the woods with my dogs.

Pets need the sights and sounds that resonate with their instincts and interaction with their guardian to be engaged with life. And our engagement with our pets enriches us.

My clients have lots of anecdotal evidence of what they see as boredom in their pets. It falls into two categories: excessive sleeping (admittedly a tough call with cats) and destructive behavior. I believe boredom inspired behavior is the main reason furniture building continues to be one of the more profitable industries in our country, along with lawn sprinkler businesses and nurseries.

My clients know the wisdom of following these three principles of good health: weight control, physical exercise and mental exercise. It's one of those simple but not easy things. It can be tempting to overfeed our pets out of love. I know it can sometimes be a challenge for guardians to get outside to exercise, and that they are always looking for ways to provide indoor exercise, both physical and mental. We all do the best we can with what we have. There may be no small irony in the mutual benefit of the bond at work here. It could be that it is our pets who exercise us, take us for walks, keep us fit and trim and keep us engaged with them – and life.

Saying Goodbye

It was my intent from the outset to have Bailee and Shilo with me to celebrate the completion of this book. But they passed, both within several months of each other, before I completed it.

Shilo was the first to leave. Her withdrawing from life had been so gradual that it became difficult to conceive of an ending, as if old age was ageless, that there would be no arrival of that final breath. We simply lived together one day at a time and I believe she would be proud of me because, after all, I had been under her and Bailee's tutelage in the art of "living in the moment."

Shilo began to worry me with a curious change in her behavior. She began to pace. Her pacing seemed to be triggered by my presence and I thought it was her way of telling me she wasn't feeling "quite right", that something was amiss. Her pacing was accompanied by the rhythmic sound of her panting, a sound that had recently taken on a raspy edge to it. And every so often she would steal a furtive glance in my direction as if to reassure herself that I had not disappeared on her.

It was disturbing to see her acting this way and I began to suspect the cause was a decline in her faculties. I noticed, too, that her sight and hearing had been steadily failing her. What troubled me most was the thought that fear might be driving her behavior. I cannot know for certain that it was, but my bond with her was strong. I trusted my intuition that was telling me my lifelong companion was frightened.

I first noticed her failing eyesight when she began to drop treats that I tossed her way. In her younger years she had no problem catching even the poorly tossed morsels, but now most fell untouched to the floor. Her pupils had first taken on the telltale grayish hue of early cataracts before slowly clouding over into a milky opacity that blurred her ability to see.

Her hearing seemed to go more suddenly. At first I had to speak more loudly to get her attention and then even a loud clap would sometimes fail to rouse her. She became more prone to being startled; I had to be careful not to approach her too quietly before touching her. More than once my touch had sent her scurrying for cover. I imagined her world as slowly folding in on itself, vision reduced to mere blurred shadows and hearing diminished to muffled sounds. I could tell by Shilo's response to my call that she was uncertain from where the sound came. She would swing her head from side to side as if trying to "catch" my presence.

Something seemed to be missing from her normal self, something beyond the failure of her senses. Shilo seemed confused. She would have periods where she would stand still, frozen, as if unsure of where she was or what it was she needed to do next. As time wore on I realized that they were the early signs of senility. I believe senility affects animals and humans in similar ways. Perhaps her uneasiness was the same kind of agitation the elderly experience when their faculties ebb and the world becomes confusing.

In any case, it was clear to me that she would need my care more than ever before. This growing dependence on me was a new phase in our relationship that I had difficulty accepting.

At first, I could not let go of the Shilo of yesteryear, still holding onto the memories of her in her prime.

I had always been a good guardian to her but my role was changing more to one of caretaker. Her ability to share life's pleasures with me was fading and I needed to accept this new "stage" in her life. I felt myself being gradually pulled into the reality of her "fading" world, preparing me for the sadness that would soon follow when her time with me would end.

There were those precious moments when Shilo would hobble over to me for solace. She would press her head against my leg and stand quietly while I massaged her ears. It was times like these when I found myself drawn into the mystery of our bond with each other. I believe that somewhere in the matrix of our bond there is a special element that makes it all possible: Shilo is a sentient creature. And therefore she has some of the same desires I have and can comprehend some of the same things, albeit to a lesser degree, or perhaps just in a different way. I think this plays a major role in her ability to bond with another sentient being of an entirely different species.

I know the word "sentient" is controversial but those of us who include pets as family members can't help but believe that they are indeed sentient creatures. Intuition, not logic, tells me so. I need no proof for its existence, I just know it is present, embedded in the bond I have with my ailing friend, Shilo. As death drew closer I was aware that our bond strengthened, sharpening my awareness of her needs, making me better able to administer to her growing dependence.

There were times when her "worrying" worsened and I would sometimes put her in her kennel with a bed of cedar shavings, where she would curl up and fall into a deep slumber. I think she liked the safety that this enclosed refuge offered her. During our final months together, I was amused to note that there was one "sense" that stubbornly refused to be taken from her by the ravages of time. My yellow Lab had retained that one sense that had served her most faithfully throughout her life: smell. It remained as sharp and keen as it was in our first walks together in the woods. That one "super" sense that always led her safely home and never once failed to bring her to her most favorite place: her food dish.

Both Bailee and Shilo retained this singular sense that seems immune to the aging process. With fully functioning noses, they continued their love for our walks into the field and forest. Nearly blind and deaf and slowed by arthritic limbs, they moved along with nose to the ground, tails beating wildly as if to announce they had once again flouted time. Their infirmities seemed to melt away leaving them young once more, their slumbering instincts reawakened by the familiar scents of a world they had known since puppyhood. Nature gave them a brief respite from the clutches of old age. It was their moment of renewal, shedding years as easily as they did their winter coats.

Late one evening, it came upon her suddenly. It was near midnight when I found Shilo standing before me laboring to breath. The look in her eyes was one of desperation. One glance at her distended belly gave me an instant diagnosis: bloat. I knew that unless she was attended to immediately she would certainly die a horribly painful death. I carried her out to my truck and headed into town for the Pet ER.

I cursed how time slowed, making my trip into town seem

interminable, even the traffic lights conspired, turning "red" whenever my truck neared an intersection. There were few cars at this late hour so I crossed against the lights. After I reached the ER, it took but a few moments before the diagnosis was confirmed. I had brought Shilo here less than a year before for the same problem, but this time the X-ray showed her bloat had taken an ominous turn – her stomach had twisted upon itself. Her only chance for life would be to take her into emergency surgery.

Her chances of making it through surgery was complicated by her advanced age, and I knew with certainty that this was the time to say goodbye. I promised myself I would be Shilo's guardian, her faithful guardian. She is old, and as she lay there on the floor, head in my lap, I knew it was time to end her suffering and not a time for heroic measures.

I was with her as she took that last breath I thought would never arrive. I was with her when her lovely dance was over. Our walks together would become memories. She had lived life well. I found myself living the history of my own book and it did not help ease the despair I fell into that night on the ER floor.

I believe Shilo's death hastened Bailee's decline. She, like Shilo, was very old – 14 years. Bailee had been suffering from Cushing's disease, a syndrome shared with their human counterparts. This chronic disease, along with Shilo's death, steepened her decline and I began to feel the growing weight of another loss looming.

Each spring I would have Bailee's winter coat trimmed by the groomers and she would return home looking sleek and shiny. I can remember her prancing though our front door in years past, acting as if she thought quite highly of herself, much more svelte than her companion, Shilo, who, after all, was just a common Labrador.

But now her wonderful coat had taken a sharp turn for the worst. Both age and Cushing's disease began attacking her hair and skin. She developed a nest of oozing sores that covered much of her body. The special sheen she wore for so many years was gone, dulled by hair turned brittle and dry. I had tried various medications and special shampoos for her Cushing's disease in an attempt to restore her coat but nothing worked. Her mottled appearance was such a sad contrast to how she looked just a year ago.

My attention to her physical appearance had distracted me from noticing that her temperament was changing. I began noticing that she was becoming "dull." Her vitality ebbed and in the weeks following Shilo's death, I noticed that she began to act as though she wasn't all there – as if her life-force was being leached out of her by age, disease, and now, death. Bailee stopped being Bailee. It was painful to recall what seemed like only yesterday that she was still so full of energy and playfulness.

Early one morning, several months after her companion had left, I had gone to the back door to call her inside. She was standing just beyond the back steps, standing on the patio, totally unresponsive to my calling her. It was as if she had become frozen, standing completely motionless, not even turning her head in my direction. She remained rooted in place as I walked over to her and placed my hand on her head. She slowly looked up at me but her stare was empty of the gentle warmness I'm accustomed to. And most unsettling was the stub of her tail failed to respond to my touch with its characteristic blur of welcoming excitement. It was difficult to look at her, so chilling to see her appear so emptied of life.

I found myself helpless to resist the dreadful thought that Bailee was trying to tell me something in the only way she could. I believe she was telling me she was ready to leave. She was giving me silent and unwanted permission to let go of her. A flood of memories crowded in on me of all the many, many clients that stood before me with tears in their eyes saying, "It's time for me to say goodbye." And now that "time" has arrived at my doorstep and I know what I must do.

I slowly bent down, gathered her gently into my arms, and carried her to my truck. She did not resist, did not object to being placed in the seat beside me, no longer rising to look out the window as I back down the driveway. Sadly, I head once again to the pet ER. This time the ride was much worse. She was my last and has protected me from the brunt of Shilo's passing. But now as she lay quietly beside me, I realized I was about to lose them both.

It's so painful to write down these thoughts, having such finality. I cannot pen my moment on the back patio with Bailee without it bringing tears to my eyes. The act of writing about my companions has had a cathartic effect on me. Human grief is personal. We each must find a way through the heartache and for me it happens during the act of writing.

I'm envious over how my granddaughter grieved. She too, is a lover of pets. For her, the grief over the loss of our two hunters came on fast and hard like a summer storm; but then, it quickly passed, washing away the core of her despair and leaving a gentle sadness in its wake. For me, acceptance does not come so easily. I muddy the waters by becoming entangled in a maze of thoughts and emotions, and it will take time before I find my way out.

I dug one grave on a knoll of a hill overlooking the fields and woods they had spent their entire life exploring. I had Shilo cremated because I did not want her taking her distended abdomen into the grave with her. I had saved her ashes so that I could place them beside Bailee's body, her lifelong companion. And I am comforted by the thought that they are together – companions unto death.

Perhaps the ultimate lesson that Bailee and Shilo taught me was to make me conscious of just how limited our time together is. Nothing lasts forever. That time revealed the fullness of the bond – the joy and the suffering – in both life and death. Becoming conscious of that limit forced me to take a closer look at death, to become more personal and more familiar with it. The wonderful irony is that as I've become less fearful of death, I've also become more available to life. The grip that death has had on me since childhood has eased.

Of course it's not my pets alone who have taught me to be less fearful of death. I've witnessed the bittersweet relief a guardian experiences at the moment of his or her suffering pet's passing. I've seen the relief that comes from deep in a person's soul when he or she knows that the struggle has ended, and, with it, the suffering. A sense of peace descends once the battle is finished. I've stood in awe whenever I witnessed these moments of struggle, and I've admired the courage and love of those who surrender the bond to death.

A Pet's Final Gift

The final gift that our pets may give us through the bond is the stories we tell about them. These stories enable us to share the love – and grief – we experience, and, in a way, define our bond with our pets.

It's a blessing for families to find refuge in storytelling, especially during the times when a pet has passed on. Grief sheds some of its ache when blended into the entirety of life's story. The bond finds renewed life in the telling of the rich stories left behind by our four-legged companions.

Humans sometimes think of death as the severing of our bond with our pets, but I don't think it's true. Death does not have the power to destroy the human-animal connection. The bond is resilient and survives death through memories. In turn, these memories can be coaxed from the quietude of our souls, given a voice, and allowed to enter into the story. The storyteller combines our voices, weaving them together word by word, until living images are created. The bond has been given a new home. What we thought was lost is found.

Family comes together in this sharing. Stories begin to emerge, and, like an old song, one spoken memory jogs loose another, and then another, until they flow around the room, joining together as the heart of this precious bond begins to take form. It is a time of reverence, and even as I struggle with the mystery of it all, I marvel at the power and grace of stories to bring healing.

Grief occurs whenever death involves a bond; suffering is the evidence of its presence. We can keep the memories of our pets alive in stories, but we cannot make up for the loss of a physical presence: the feel of a cold, moist nose pressed against a hand, of fur running between our fingers, of the soothing hum of a purr, of a sharp bark reminding us it's dinner time, a companion to share our walks, a body to fill the empty room with presence, a feeling of purpose as we care for them. These are gone, replaced by the deafening silence of emptiness, and we grieve. The loneliness will linger, as will the pain and sadness, but these will lessen over time, helped by the telling of stories.

The unfolding of the story is especially important when children are part of the bond. There is sanctity to the grieving process that needs to be protected from judgment – a place where remembrances are safe to share, a setting where acceptance encourages a child the risk of being heard. It could be a time for them to speak of sadness and joy, of fear and confusion over this stranger called death, a time to encourage their sharing, to honor their feelings, to accept them as unconditionally as their pets accepted them. I shudder remembering a young woman telling me of a time in her childhood when she was grieving over the loss of the family pet. Her father, tiring of her tears, yelled, "For crying out loud, get over it! It's just a pet." And it only deepened her pain.

Perhaps it is here within the circle of sharing where a child can overcome the fear of asking their secreted questions: "Why did he have to die? Where is Fido now? Will he come back? Is he still in the ground? Will I see him again? Do pets go to heaven? Why did you have to put Fido to sleep*?"

---

*A word of caution about the word sleep: it can be scary for a child to "go to sleep" after a pet has been "put to sleep" from which there is no awakening.

Some of us will struggle more than others to answer these questions. We struggle more if, when we were children, our questions about death went unanswered or dismissed with an unhelpful cliché. There may not have been a time to share our grief over the loss of a childhood pet, and so we find ourselves uncomfortable and unsure of just how to undo the silence when a pet has passed away and our child is looking to us for a way to navigate this strange world of death and grief. Children need to enter into a story to help quell the uncertainties and fears inherent in loss and to find a place where they can share precious memories and maybe a sad, sweet laugh at a pet's unforgettable foibles. I would suggest that the death of a family pet can encourage discussion about topics that are otherwise too difficult for children to broach – including their own deaths.

The following passage by Albert Schweitzer expresses the alchemy of how I believe a pet's death can bring meaning to life.

"We must all become familiar with the thought of death if we want to grow into really good people. We need not think of it every day or every hour. But when the path of life leads us to some vantage point where the scene around us fades away and we contemplate the distant view right to the end, let us not close our eyes.

Let us pause for a moment, look at the distant view, and then carry on. Thinking about death in this way produces love for life. When we are familiar with death, we accept each week, each day, as a gift. Only if we are able thus to accept life bit-by-bit, does it become precious."

Could this be our pet's final gift to us, the gift of making us more familiar with the thought of death, of giving it a voice within the story? I would like to think that the loss of a pet might be providential by encouraging us to return to that dusty place where we have swept away our thoughts about death, a place where we would rather not go.

Stories give us a way to go there, not only to accept the finality of loss – the wound that will always be with us – but also to experience and move though grief to a new life where memory lives in story.

Breaking a legacy of silence that sometimes surrounds death can help us through life's vicissitudes, and, like when we sense our pet's life is nearing the end we are given an opportunity to become more "familiar with the thought of death", to "pause for a moment" and not "close our eyes". Then, over the time surrounding death we give voice to our grief to help soften the harsh edges of suffering. It is not yet finished. We are called not to thoughts of death but to those of life...inviting us to re-live those precious moments of joy and laughter. In this way death is denied the final word. Even those who are not ready to share their "moments" can visit them in the quietude of self-reflection. Our pets have offered us their final gift, helping us to "grow into really good people". I think Albert Schweitzer would agree.

I am struck by the resiliency of the human spirit during times of grief. I have been to a number of human memorial services, and the ones that stand out in my mind are the ones where humor weaves its way into the life of the departed one. It seems to me that sorrow has a special affinity for humor in times of suffering. They come together in a way that is protective, where humor keeps sorrow from deepening into despair. I have often seen these "tears of laughter" coursing down the cheeks of those left behind as they recall some poignant memory of times gone by.

I am grateful for our human capacity to create humor out of memories of times when it went missing. Somehow, events of the past that brought anger and frustration are mysteriously transformed into levity.

I remember a client once telling me about a time that serves as a wonderful example. Shortly after his pet Smoky, a Shetland sheepdog, had passed, he was reminiscing with his daughter about the time Smoky stole the Thanksgiving turkey off the dinner table. The family's grandmother had flown in to spend this special holiday with her loved ones, but now the meal was missing its signature dish. They spent the remainder of their holiday evening at my clinic with a vomiting pet.

"Remember how mad you were that day!" the daughter laughed as she spoke to her dad. "Your face was so red you scared Grandma almost to death!" "Yes, I remember," he laughed, "but at the time it wasn't a bit funny." I think laughing was their way of completely forgiving Smokey for his indiscretions, not just for eating the turkey but also for all his transgressions. All the difficult times seemed to be wrapped up in one long, hearty laugh. Maybe laughter was the way for them to forgive themselves for being so angry and upset when their pet failed to be what he could not be. Putting a dog unattended in a room filled with the aroma of a freshly baked turkey is like leaving a child alone with a jar full of freshly baked cookies.

So many clients, so many memories. Someone recalls a story, and heaven knows pets provide us with a storehouse of rich animal memories, and we begin to laugh. Stories of steaks disappearing from the barbecue, ice cream cones stolen right out of a child's hand, a toy chewed into tiny bits and pieces, a fishhook finding its way from the tackle box into a curious tongue, screen doors shredded for the tenth time, those frantic retreats into the sanctity of a dark closet to escape the menacing rumble of a sudden summer storm or the cacophony of yet another Fourth of July. Humor seeps into these stories as a way of letting go. Our laughter is not the kind you hear from those trying to flee from pain; rather it is the kind that comes from deep within the pain.

When we reflect on times gone by through the prism of grief, we discover that our thoughts have been mysteriously softened. When upon all those times we tried to control our pet's behavior, when we look carefully at our futile efforts to tame the maverick in him or her, we suddenly realize our pet's free-spirited nature is what we miss the most. We find ourselves accepting our pet just the way she or he was. I like to think of this acceptance as a place of refuge, as an extension of what our pets have given us all the days of their lives: unconditional acceptance.

And thus we arrive at our pet's final gift. I call the gift "The Great Exchange". We surrender our reluctance to accept death's arrival in exchange for the lifetime of memories they gave to us. Storytelling is a wonderful way to become "familiar with the thought of death" when we share our grief with others. Through our remembrances we can re-experience those "living" moments, those precious "bits" of our pet's life that brought us joy and laughter… and yes, frustration. Their death also gives us an opportunity to forgive ourselves for being too human in our inability to accept them as they accepted us: just the way we are. I do not suggest this "exchange" is easy...it takes courage. I have witnessed these acts of courage throughout my years of practice. And I have been humbled. As I look back on my profession and reflect on how I handled those heartbreaking moments of losing a pet, I realize that there was a point beyond which I could not go. I could help a client understand the nature of a pet's ailment, clarify the confusion by using familiar words as substitutes for our medical jargon, and this might have helped prepare a client for the pet's passing. I could share my own stories and be present to hear theirs. But I believed that I must also respect the sanctity of their thoughts, especially those of a spiritual nature, however different they might be from my own. Death challenges our spiritual convictions – making us think about life after death and whether we will find our pet in that afterlife.

Over time, I have become more familiar with the thought of death, but I have not arrived at a place where I am without fear. Death will always carry a sense of mystery for me, arousing not only my curiosity but also awakening what I would call a respectful touch of misgiving.

I no longer condemn myself for not finding complete comfort and peace with this matter, and after many years of helping others through the process of ending a pet's life, I still think of myself as a pilgrim. I have accepted how little I really know, and how often my answer to deeper questions about death is "It's a mystery." But I am certain about one thing: pets, even in their dying, help us to become better people to live life more fully.

If Pets Could Write

If Pets could write about the bond – and the pain we feel when it ends – what would they say? It is only out of hubris that I could even presume to know what goes on in the mind of a pet. It surely is a mystery, a profound mystery. But I feel compelled to give my best guess – I've been their faithful doctor for so long; just let me guess what a pet might say. I offer these letters to readers as a vehicle for consolation – and confirmation of the power of the bond to enrich our lives.

Dear (guardian's name),

It appears to you as if my time has passed so very quickly, but the pace of time is as it should be – for my years are not your years. You think I am rushing through life, but that's only from your perspective. For me, time just is.

You must understand how much I loved being with you through my years. I felt comforted. I had food when I was hungry, warmth when I was cold, shelter from the elements, and most of all I had you and you were always there. You were never stingy with your gentle stroking or with those walks down our country lane when the evening sun loomed low.

So now my time is ending; my legs have weakened—I cannot stand. There is some internal signal that tells me that if I could, I would find some small den to crawl into, curl myself into a tight ball and drift away. So please don't try to keep me on this side of life, away from where I am ready to go. I do not fear death as humans do. We are born, we grow, and then we die. And that is as it should be. In fact, we don't even have a word for death. The closest I can get to a meaning for death is simply "as it should be."

Don't feel guilty about helping me to die. Please don't keep me suspended in this state where I can no longer rise, where I soil my bedding, and where my rest is more an endless ache. This tells me it is time to go. I sense that I am not well, that my time has been used up, and now I must go to another place. I go with no misgivings, sadness, fear or thought of what comes next. I only know this simple thing: it is time for me to go. If I linger, I will suffer in a physical sense, but you will suffer in ways that I cannot imagine. You will feel dread, anxiety, guilt, shame, heartache, fear and anguish. Remember, these are your feelings and you must not think they're mine – for if you do, you do not know me.

I am tired now, so tired. When I can no longer be what I have been, when I do things against my nature, I feel only that something is not right, and so I tell you: it's all right to let me go.

Goodbye,
Your faithful companion,
(Your pet's name)

Reply

Dear (your pet's name),

Thank you so much for your letter to me. I have read it many times, and feel I owe you this apology.

Because of your words, I more fully understand that the nature of my own suffering is different from yours. I, too, feel the pain of aging. My hips do ache, and I know that the future will bring other kinds of physical pain. What you taught me in your letter is that I must deal with my emotional pain and see it as mine and not yours. I want you to be more human than what nature has created. I find it difficult to accept our differences, but I am grateful that you do not suffer in the ways we humans must. I read your list over, and the one feeling that most describes how I feel about your impending death is anguish. For me, anguish is so strong a feeling that it becomes physical as an ache deep inside – an ache that makes me want to hold on to you.

To a lesser degree I feel guilt. I know I want to keep you out of that den where you want to "curl up and drift away," but if I am to help you die, I must take you to a pet hospital and ask the vet to put you down. The thought of this is so difficult that I can't find the words to describe the depth of my despair. "How do I end something I love?" I ask myself. I've found the answer to be simple but painful: by suffering. This suffering will be created out of a strange paradox: it is because I love you that I end your life. The only way this will happen is for me to suffer. I must overcome my own need for you to live so that I can attend to your needs. When I put your needs above my own, I see more clearly my responsibilities as your trusted guardian.

But when is the time right? How will I know you are ready? I asked that question of our veterinarian. He didn't answer right away, but after some time he looked into my eyes and said that the correct time comes out of my suffering, and I must trust in this. He promised he would do his best to help me understand where you are in your ailment and promised to be there for me as my guardian as I am yours. I will suffer most in overcoming my need to keep you with me. I hope I can be worthy of that suffering.

Your trusted guardian and best friend,
(Your name)

www.ingramcontent.com/pod-product-compliance
Lightning Source LLC
Chambersburg PA
CBHW072340300426
44109CB00043B/1973